Oscar Francisco Gonzales Gamarra
Juan Pablo N. de Guzmán Zamalloa
Nicolás León Pérez León Pérez

Most common etiology of trigeminal neuralgia

Oscar Francisco Gonzales Gamarra
Juan Pablo N. de Guzmán Zamalloa
Nicolás León Pérez León Pérez

Most common etiology of trigeminal neuralgia

In patients seen in Cusco from January 2019 to August 2022

ScienciaScripts

Cover image: www.ingimage.com

This book is a translation from the original published under ISBN 978-613-9-05126-7.

Publisher:
Sciencia Scripts
is a trademark of
Dodo Books Indian Ocean Ltd. and OmniScriptum S.R.L publishing group

120 High Road, East Finchley, London, N2 9ED, United Kingdom
Str. Armeneasca 28/1, office 1, Chisinau MD-2012, Republic of Moldova, Europe
Managing Directors: Ieva Konstantinova, Victoria Ursu
info@omniscriptum.com

Printed at: see last page
ISBN: 978-620-8-37025-1

Contents

Dedication

To Dr. Oscar Francisco Gonzales Gamarra, as a tribute in life, to this eminent neurologist, participant of this study, for his dedication, ethics and service for so many decades as a specialist physician; all my admiration, gratitude and respect; as well as inspiring me to be a better researcher, professional and person.

To my family who, from my grandparents onwards, have always instilled in me the gift of service.

To my friends Blga. Erica Escalante Pompilla and C.D. Juan Jairo Pinedo Portugal, for encouraging me to represent Peru scientifically abroad.

To my friends Pedro Efrain Salas Cardenas, Jose Antonio Valverde Ellera, Silvia Dapueto and Maria Cecilia Petralia, for being people who, in spite of living in other latitudes, they are always there.

Acknowledgement

To Dr. Victor Edwin Ore Montalvo for being first and foremost a great person, professional and advisor of this thesis.

To the Hospital Adolfo Guevara Velasco- EsSalud Cusco, for giving me the opportunity to grow as a researcher.

To C.D. Iriana Pena Manrique and Nicolas Leon Perez, for agreeing to be part of this research.

To my statistician Mg. Mayra Alejandra Perez Parra, for being my right hand in this scientific study.

"He who does not live to serve does not serve to live". (Matthew 20: 27-29)

Summary

The trigeminal nerve originates from the ophthalmic (V1), maxillary (V2) and mandibular (V3) branches, whose trigeminal neuralgia (TN) causes pain when chewing and manipulating gums, forcing a visit to the dentist before the neurologist or neurosurgeon; topographically, it affects branches V1 4%; V2 23%; V3 15%; V1 and V2 16.5%; V2 and V3 32%. ***Aim: To*** identify the most common aetiology of TN in patients seen at EsSalud Cusco from January 2019 to August 2022. ***Metodo:*** Non-experimental type, qualitative, quantitative, retrospective and cross-sectional approach; the sample, 127 datas of clinical histories diagnosed with TN, in Neurology, Neurosurgery and Dentistry of the Hospital EsSalud-Cusco; the instrument the data collection form, the unit of analysis the clinical history and the method the indirect observation; the most common aetiology and TN, measured on data collection sheets, by expert record by means of an evaluator; the scores diagnosed for X, according to predisposing and aetiological factors and for Y by types of TN and pain scales; finally the type of analysis, descriptive statistics. ***Results**:* Most common aetiological variable: predisposing factor, sex 79.5% and aetiological factor, unknown aetiology 55.1%. Trigeminal neuralgia variable: Type of TN, idiopathic 34.6%; severe pain 59.1% according to VAS scale. ***Conclusion:*** Predisposing sex and etiology unknown etiology is the most common etiology of TN, affecting branches V1, V2 and V3 at 19.9% in patients seen in EsSalud Cusco from 2019 to August 2022.

Keywords: pain; most common aetiology; aetiological factors; predisposing factors; trigeminal nerve; trigeminal neuralgia; neurosurgery; neurology; neurology; dentistry; type of TN

Subject areas: Endodontics; neurology; neurology; dentistry; neurosurgery; endodontics

Introduction

The present study on the "Most common aetiology of trigeminal neuralgia (TN) in patients seen in EsSalud Cusco from January 2019 to August 2022" has the purpose of informing dentists of the importance of interconsultations with the neurologist in situations of non-odontogenic pain such as TN. In this regard, Antonaci, et al. (2020) point out that this procedure benefits patients, as quality of life is seriously affected (1).

Research into all aspects of TN (natural history, clinical picture, diagnosis, treatment and prognosis) is relevant (2). At the same time, the picture of atypical orofacial pain is highlighted (3).

In the National Hospital Adolfo Guevara Velasco - EsSalud Cusco, there is a lack of data on the prevalence and incidence of trigeminal neuralgia; there is little communication between the dentist and the disciplines of neurology and neurosurgery regarding this condition.

Specifying the problem, the central question of the work is ^What is the most common etiology of trigeminal neuralgia in patients treated in EsSalud Cusco from January 2019 to August 2022?

That is why the present study highlights the central objective of identifying the most common aetiology of trigeminal neuralgia in patients treated in EsSalud Cusco from January 2019 to August 2022.

This research project is structured in three chapters. Chapter I "Approach of the study" describes the problem of the study, as well as the formulation of the problem, the justification, the objectives and the hypotheses. In chapter II "Theoretical framework" some theoretical and conceptual clarifications are developed, as well as the most common aetiology and genesis of trigeminal neuralgia. In chapter III "Methodology", the operationalization of the variables, the sample and the methods of the study are carried out. Finally, chapter IV "Results and discussion" contains the statistical part, the findings and discussions corresponding to this scientific study. Additionally, the conclusions of the research, as well as the respective recommendations, bibliographical references and annexes.

CHAPTER 1

APPROACH TO THE STUDY

1.1 Problematic Situation

Worldwide, most patients present with a normal physical and neurological examination, lacking reliable biomarkers for the disease (2). It has been shown that genetic predisposition in trigeminal neuralgia (TN) may involve multiple genes and/or downstream products, such as ion channels, thus TN may be multifactorial (4), and is more frequent than previously assumed (1). In this regard, Boto (2010) highlights that the incidence is 4 per 100,000 inhabitants (5). There is a possibility that the new SARS-CoV-2 coronavirus is a secondary aetiology of TN (6). Thus, in one case report, a patient was treated for odontalgia, when in fact he was suffering from acute trigeminal neuralgia, post Pfizer-BioNtech SARS-CoV-2 vaccine (7). In another scenario, a 49-year-old patient developed trigeminal neuralgia (TN) with a 10-year history of acute, dull, constant, mechanical-sensory stimulus pain in the third branch of the trigeminal nerve as a result of a chronic dental infection in the left upper premolar area (8). Demonstrating that there is a need for greater understanding of the disease by dentists and better management of patients for timely and correct treatment, without sacrificing any teeth. Therefore, the onus is on neurosurgeons/neurologists to disseminate knowledge about proper diagnosis and treatment modalities (9).

At the Latin American level, the mastery and information of this physiopathology would help stomatologists, neurologists and neurosurgeons to differentiate between typical and atypical TN and odontogenic pain (10). Thus, for example, a 73 year old patient with facial discomfort, whose real diagnosis was TN type I, was insistently subjected to root canals at 22, 23 and 25, the latter with apicoectomy, as well as exodontia at 24 and 26 (11). As for the age factor, it manifests itself between 50 and 90 years of age, with the female sex being the most recurrent in 67% and 33% male; according to topography, it manifests itself more in the maxillary branch (V2) unilaterally in the left facial area in 72% of cases; the degree of pain is severe in 47% of cases according to the Valleix test (3). Finally, it has been observed that the "post-COVID neurological syndrome" represents a challenge for the clinical neurologist because of the multiple manifestations of the central and peripheral nervous system with musculoskeletal and neuropsychiatric symptoms, without a classic semiology, for example: intense and constant headache, insomnia, anxiety and unexplained depression in patients with no previous history (12).

At the national level, the most affected patients are women (76.7%), with the most affected side being the right (59.5%) in the maxillary branch (33.23%) (13).

Among the different causes that may be causing this problem, we have detected the following: Lack of diffusion of neurologists and neurosurgeons about TN to the dental profession, lack of information of the dentist about TN and recurrence of the patient to the dental office instead of going to the neurological office for an apparently dental pain.

If no conscious action is taken, the patient subjected to a sustained NT crisis over time without being properly diagnosed and treated "could lead to suicides" (14). Likewise, dental services would continue to provide care without referral to a specialist, leaving patients mutilated in the mouth. Above all, dentists should consider the VAS pain scale of atypical odontalgia (OA) when confronted with odontalgia without a reasonable organic cause and avoid unnecessary dental procedures (11).

The existing problem will have implications in professional training, therefore, this research aims to generate knowledge of the problem of the lack of knowledge on how to determine the origin of odontogenic and non-odontogenic pain, taking advantage of interconsultations with neurologists in our locality or making use of social networks for video consultations, so that all the specialists involved in the area (neurologists, neurosurgeons and dentists) benefit so that they can work together and especially for the benefit of the patient. Finally, it should be analysed how many patients with non-odontogenic pain come to the dental surgery every month.

1.2 Formulation of the problem

In accordance with the empirical foundation and observation of the phenomenon in reality, the general problem is posed in the following terms:

1.2.1 General problem

/What is the most common aetiology of trigeminal neuralgia in patients seen at Es salud Cusco from January 2019 to August 2022?

1.2.2 Specific problems

a) /Is there a relation between TN and *age* in patients seen in EsSalud Cusco from January 2019 to August 2022?

b) /What is the relationship between TN and *sex* in patients seen in EsSalud Cusco from January 2019 to August 2022?

c) /What is the relation between TN and *covid* in patients treated in EsSalud Cusco from January 2019 to August 2022?

d) /What is the relationship between NT and *genetics* in patients treated in EsSalud Cusco from January 2019 to August 2022?

e) /What is the relation between TN and *tumours* in patients treated in EsSalud Cusco from January 2019 to August 2022?

1.3 Theoretical justification

The present study is *important* because its results will contribute to the areas of Neurology, Neurosurgery and Dentistry; improving educational, medical, dental and social practices, which is of great importance for the teachers of the Neurology, Neurosurgery and Endodontics courses.

The work is of *scientific relevance,* as it makes an important contribution to research (15). Since this is one of the fields of Neurology, Neurosurgery and Dentistry that needs special care and treatment by those involved, it will serve as a contribution to other scientific and technical purposes, especially in the medical field.

It is of *social relevance*, because according to Boto (2010), it affects 1 person per 100,000 inhabitants and more women than men (5).

1.4 Practical justification

It presents *singularity, novelty and originality* since there are few updated studies on trigeminal neuralgia.

It is topical because COVID is one of the probable causes of trigeminal neuralgia (16).

It presents *viability and feasibility* to be investigated, because it investigates information contained in the institution to be studied.

There is a *personal interest*, as there is a special preference for the study of the most common aetiology of trigeminal neuralgia, due to the frequent cases of odontalgia in the dental office.

1.5 Objectives

1.5.1. General objective

To identify the most common aetiology of trigeminal neuralgia in patients treated at EsSalud Cusco from January 2019 to August 2022.

1.5.2. Specific objectives

a) To determine the relationship between TN and age in patients seen in EsSalud Cusco from January 2019 to August 2022.

b) To compare the relationship between TL and gender in patients seen in EsSalud Cusco from January 2019 to August 2022.

c) To associate the relationship between TN and COVID in patients treated at EsSalud Cusco from January 2019 to August 2022.

d) To establish the relationship between TN and genetics in patients treated at EsSalud Cusco from January 2019 to August 2022.

e) To describe the relationship between TN and tumours in patients treated at EsSalud Cusco from January 2019 to August 2022.

1.6 Hypothesis

1.6.1 General hypothesis

HGA. There is a more common aetiology of trigeminal neuralgia in patients treated in EsSalud Cusco from January 2019 to August 2022.

HGO. There is no common etiology of trigeminal neuralgia in patients seen in EsSalud Cusco from January 2019 to August 2022.

1.6.2. Specific hypotheses

1.6.2.1 Specific scenario 01

Ha. There is a relationship between TN and age in patients seen in EsSalud Cusco from January 2019 to August 2022.

Ho. There is no relationship between TN and age in patients seen in EsSalud Cusco from January 2019 to August 2022.

1.6.2.2 Specific scenario 02

Ha. There is a relationship between TN and gender in patients seen in EsSalud Cusco from January 2019 to August 2022.

Ho. There is no relationship between TN and gender in patients seen in EsSalud Cusco from January 2019 to August 2022.

1.6.2.2 Specific Hypothesis 03

Ha. There is a relationship between TN and COVID in patients seen in EsSalud Cusco from January 2019 to August 2022.

Ho. There is no relationship between TN and COVID in patients seen in EsSalud Cusco from January 2019 to August 2022.

1.6.2.3 Specific Hypothesis 04

Ha. Existe relación entre la NT y la genetica en pacientes atendidos en EsSalud Cusco desde enero del 2019 hasta agosto del 2022.

Ho. There is no relationship between TN and genetics in patients seen in EsSalud Cusco from January 2019 to August 2022.

1.6.2.4 Specific Hypothesis 05

Ha. There is a relationship between TN and tumours in patients treated at EsSalud Cusco from January 2019 to August 2022.

Ho. There is no relationship between TN and tumours in patients seen in EsSalud Cusco from January 2019 to August 2022.

CHAPTER 2

THEORETICAL FRAMEWORK

2.1 Philosophical or epistemological framework of research

Describing the philosophical or epistemological framework in this research, on the variables Most Common Aetiology as variable X and Trigeminal Neuralgia as variable Y, emerges from the curiosity to determine the relationship that exists between these with their respective dimensions; and thus to be able to understand the preponderance of these and the changes that could be given in the formative, professional and patient field.

While Ontology, Neurology and Neurosurgery are intertwined in the philosophical stance of medica. A fuzzy boundary persists (Ackroyd and Fleetwood, 2000), as a model: "Substituting the epistemological question 'How to understand what is found' for the ontological approach 'What is found'? Humanly we would deduce that what is present is given by our definitions or conceptions. A pallidly erroneous deduction".

Therefore, the conception of the process of training-improving the quality of life of patients requires some elements to be considered, such as predisposing and aetiological factors, in addition to the classes of TN and their pain scales, in relation to their corresponding dimensions, without forgetting the health, latitude and geographical context.

Learning according to the reality of those involved encompasses scientific, technical and ethical points, which intersect valuationally and epistemologically (Diaz, 2008).

Therefore, it is suggested to take into consideration those proposals through other scholars, which help to understand the occurrence of certain facts, manifested according to the context in which they are found, creating confrontations, which the researcher must overcome by choosing theories with a panoramic vision, arriving at a specific approach to that which is to be demonstrated. *In this framework, Popper (1934) refers that "the method of chrtically contrasting theories and of choosing them, considering the results obtained in their contrast (...). Once a new idea has been provisionally presented, whether it is an anticipation, a hypothesis, a theoretical system or whatever is desired, conclusions are drawn by logical deduction, comparing them with each other and with other relevant statements, in order to find logical relations (equivalence, deductibility, compatibility or incompatibility, etc.) that exist between them" (p.8).*

In the present investigation, the computerised data of the patients showed intense pain, mostly triggered by harmless movements and currently without access to Magnetic Resonance Imaging (MRI).

From the above mentioned, the most relevant previous studies are considered (Vazques, 2020), who maintains that it develops more in the female public over 60 years of age and with a right facial side reach.

Indeed, Lara (2021), manifests itself in the female public over 50 years of age, with trigger zones resulting from demyelination.

Dentists, neurologists and neurosurgeons should be inspired to take the greatest possible care of trigeminal neuralgia; therefore, in order to achieve greater knowledge, encourage training between these disciplines.

"The student of dentistry and human medicine must have a basis of knowledge about Trigeminal Neuralgia, (Cargua et al., 2017), for example: a correct diagnosis leads to success in treatment. By fully complying with the parameters, the results will undoubtedly be favourable for the patient, as well as for the training of the student and the orientation of the patient".

2.2 Background to the research

a) At the national level

Tragodara (2020). TN or tic doloreux is a very painful disease, which, to avoid confusion, headaches or other conditions should be ruled out; it is currently supported by imaging; however, if not treated properly, it can lead to stress at work, social, psychological and even suicide (17).

Vasquez (2020). A total of 163 medical records from Neurology, Neurosurgery and Dentistry were examined, with data taken from a data collection form, taking into account age, sex, injured facial area and trigeminal branch, whose values were uploaded to tables and bar graphs. TN was triggered more among people between 60 and 69 years of age, more in women (76.7%), and unilaterally on the right side (59.5%), with the V2 branch being the most affected (33.23%), and because if we are not careful, we can avoid suicides due to malpractice (14).

b) At the international level

Boto (2010). TN is still an unknown pathological entity, even poorly managed by specialists. It occurs over the age of 50 and around 63 years, according to some authors it is more frequent in men (1.2:1) and for others more frequent in women. The annual incidence is about 4 per 100,000 inhabitants and it is rarely genetic. It generally affects the right hemiarch to 60% of cases, 39% manifest on the left side and 1% bilaterally with alternating pain occurring mainly in cases of multiple sclerosis, which is why 18% of patients with bilateral TN have this pathology. Likewise, the V2 and V3 branches are the most affected, with 42% of cases, the V2 branch alone with 20%, the V3 branch alone with 17% and V1 and V2 together with 14%, and V1, V2 and V3 with 5% and V1 alone with 2%.

TN rarely presents as trigeminal status or rapid succession of tic-like spasms, triggered by any stimulus, but intravenous phenytoin is very effective. It can be divided into primary, idiopathic or essential and secondary or symptomatic (5).

Von Eckardstein and Veit Rohde (2015). TN is commonly triggered by chewing and manipulation of the gums. Therefore, patients are likely to consult their dentist when it first presents before being referred to a neurologist or neurosurgeon. Of 51 patients; two-thirds reported being pain free; forty-one patients (82%) initially consulted their dentist; of these, 27 received invasive dental treatment for pain syndrome, including extractions, root canals and implants. Of 98 local dentists contacted, 51 responded, and three-quarters felt competent to assess trigeminal neuralgia. A high percentage of patients who are treated surgically for trigeminal neuralgia first consult their dentist and receive possibly unwarranted dental treatment. Differential diagnoses include odontogenic pain syndromes, as well as atypical orofacial pain. The current literature acknowledges the difficulties in correctly diagnosing trigeminal neuralgia, but seems to underestimate the extent (3).

Alcantara and Sanchez (2016). The incidence of TN is 413%, initially as a pharmacological treatment (carbamazepine 100mg- twice daily, Oxcarbazepine 300mg- twice daily, Baclofen 5mg- three times daily, gabapentin 100mg- three times daily, pregabalin 75mg once a night, lamotrigine 25mg- once daily, phenytoin 50mg- 3 times daily, topiramate 25mg- once a night dose for 7 days and then increase for 1 to 2 weeks in doses of 25-50mg twice a day, levetiracetam 250mg- twice daily); However, the non-resolution by medication leads to surgery, either open or conservative percutaneous, the latter being effective; however, its recurrence leads to a preference for vascular micro-decompression. The hope for improvement in therapeutic perspectives rests clearly on the novel procedures of radiofrequency application. Radiofrequency thermocoagulation is effective against pain in 97% of cases, with recurrence at half year of 25% and persistence of pain at decade of 52.3%; its complications are facial hypoaesthesia 1-9% and corneal anaesthesia 0-17% (18).

Alcantara and Gonzales (2017). Discernment to get NT right is terminologically weak and interferes with the relationship between the researcher, the treating physician and the patient. For this reason, the American Academy of Neurology (AAN) developed a new taxonomy with diagnostic accuracy criteria, with a classification system for neuropathic pain, created to be applied in diagnostic and treatment decisions (19).

Gossweiler (2018). Major autohaemotherapy is one of the methods of systemic administration of medical oxygen/ozone (MOZO) that can be applied to treat conditions resulting from chronic oxidative stress. This case report describes the application of major autohemotherapy, 3 sessions for 14 days prior to exodontia of tooth 36 to facilitate resolution of TN, with no symptoms at the 4-month follow-up, as a result of a chronic dental infection in that tooth in a 49-year-old female patient with a 10-year history of acute, dull, constant mechanical and sensory stimulation of the third branch of the trigeminal nerve (20).

Grin et al. (2018). Through a complete examination that includes CT, MRI and laboratory, the root canal of the affected teeth is avoided and the pharmacological intake of carbamazepine is then started. It should not be forgotten that this pathology presents as odontogenic pain, so it is urgent for stomatologists to be aware of its symptomatology. In order to avoid cases such as this 73 year old patient, who underwent root canal treatment in 22, 23 and 25, the latter with apicoectomy, as well as exodontia in 24 and 26, when the real diagnosis was TN type I (13).

Antonaci et al. (2020). They recruited 102 patients, mostly women in an F:M ratio of 2.64:1. Eighty-six percent of patients consulted a physician at the first attacks of pain. The specialists consulted before diagnosis of TN were: primary care physicians (PCP) 43.1%, dentists 30.4%, otolaryngologists 3.9%, neurosurgeons 3.9%, neurologists or headache specialists 14.7%, others 8%. The final diagnosis was made by a neurologist or headache specialist 85.3%, and the mean interval between disease onset and diagnosis by a specialist was 10.8 ± 21.2 months. The "diagnostic delay" was 7.2 ± 12.5 months and diagnostic errors were found at the first consultation in 42.1% of cases. Instrumental and laboratory investigations were performed in 93.1% of the patients before the final diagnosis of TN. The misdiagnoses were: dental problems 37.48 %, including odontalgia, periodontal abscess, caries, dental granulomas; sinusitis 14.3%; unspecified facial pain 9.1%; unspecified headache 7.8%; migraine 6.5%; cluster headache 5.2%; temporomandibular joint dysfunction 3.9%; glaucoma tension headache 1.3%, otitis 1.3%; tonsillitis 1.3%. With proper diagnosis, treatment was carbamazepine 80.3%, gabapentinoid drugs 11.7%, topiramate 2%, lamotrigine 2%; oxacarbazepine 1%, methylprednisolone 1%, opioids 1%, antidepressants 1%. In short, TN has typical features and is well defined by the available international diagnostic criteria. However, it is under-diagnosed and under-treated. Therefore, there is a need to improve neurological knowledge in order to recognise the clinical picture of TN in a timely manner and to adhere appropriately to specific guidelines. This may result in a favourable outcome for patients, whose quality of life is often severely affected (1).

Ayele et al. (2020). The age group of the 61 participants ranged from 21 to 78 years; 50.8% were male, 41% had a history of dental extractions on the involved side, while 68.9% reported involvement of the right facial side, where the most common branch was the mandibular 47.5%; (90.2%) of the patients met criteria for classic TN and 9.8% had symptomatic TN. Most participants reported mixed types of pain, such as burning, lancinating and electric shock-like. A well-defined trigger zone was identified in one third (36%) of cases. Carbamazepine was the most commonly prescribed drug with a median dose of 600 mg (RIQ: 400 - 1000 mg). Two thirds of patients reported prominent satisfaction. The mean (± SD) dose of carbamazepine used to control pain was significantly higher among those with a history of tooth extraction compared to those without a history of tooth extraction (736 ± 478.6 mg vs. 661.1 ± 360.4 mg, respectively, T = - 2.06, p = 0.04 95% CI -213.41 to -2.98). A statistically significant number of patients with single-branch involvement reported outstanding satisfaction with their treatment compared to those with more than one branch involvement (95% CI 1.3-3.8: p = 0.006) (8).

De Laat (2020). In order not to confuse odontogenic pain with non-odontogenic pain (myofascial, trigeminal neuropathy, as well as painful post-traumatic trigeminal neuropathic pain, orofacial neurovascular pain, cardiac and paranasal sinus disease). A good systemic HC with adequate anamnesis, detailed dental, periodontal, and intraoral examination and a general orofacial radiography are necessary. Finally, if the case warrants it, further examination techniques should be used (21).

Jaramillo and Mendoza (2020). Due to its unknown cause, it is essential to have a specialist medical consultation in order to rule out systemic diseases such as diabetes and arterial hypertension. Given that, it is a chronic alteration of intense pain of the V cranial nerve in both motor and sensitive portions; from 2015 to 2019 thanks to the statistical data of the dental area of the Teodoro Maldonado Carbo hospital, were tabulated absolute and relative values, plotted in tables of frequencies and percentages, identifying 39 patients with TN, which reported according to group: Age, (50-90 years) 68% or 17 females; gender, 67% or 26 females, and 33% or 13 males; locality, (sinister facial area) 72% or 28 cases; degree of pain, severe unilateral (maxillary branch or V2 on Valleix examination) 47% or 28 patients (22).

Tripathi et al. (2020). To assess whether patients underwent root canal treatment for undiagnosed TN, out of 187 patients, 117 patients participated. About 55.5% of the patients had odontalgia and 65.8% visited the dentist. About 41.8% of patients underwent a dental procedure; 18.8% had worsening pain, while 8.5% had some partial improvement. About 19.6% also underwent root canal treatment, while 6.8% had a nerve block. An average of 1.6 teeth were extracted per person. Seventy-one percent of patients were satisfied with Gamma Knife radiosurgery for TL at a median follow-up of 49 months. Ultimately, there is a need for better understanding of the disease among dentists and patients for timely and correct treatment without undergoing exodontia. Therefore, the onus is on neurosurgeons/neurologists to disseminate knowledge about proper diagnosis and treatment modalities (10).

Bara et al. (2021). Trigeminal neuralgia, or in French tic douloureux, is a painful condition of particular severity, although technically a neuropathic pain, most sources include it among the wide range of atypical headaches and facial pains. It is not uncommon for patients to be passed from one specialist to another (including dentists) and sometimes undergo unnecessary and ineffective dental treatments such as root canals and extractions, contributing to their daily ailment. As a treatment, carbamazepine has some anticholinergic effects; discovered in 1962 it changed the natural history of the disease; four years later it was marketed as Tegretol, with enthusiastic results. Of course, surgery has made remarkable advances: Janetta's microvascular decompression, focusing on Gasser's ganglion, from the hypotheses of demyelination to the "switching on" of models due to injured and hyperexcitable axons (23).

Duran and Duran (2021). Of 5070 neurological patients, 3280 were female (64.7%) and 1790 were male (35.3%); 237 of these patients presented with post-COVID neurological manifestations (4.67%). 151 were female (2.97%), 86 were male (1.69%). Forty-one percent had CNS involvement (headache, vertigo, seizures, memory disorders, tremor), 57% PNS involvement (paraesthesia, weakness, painful polyneuropathy, trigeminal neuralgia), 45% musculoskeletal involvement (myalgia, polyarthralgia) and 35% neuropsychiatric involvement (anxiety, depression, insomnia). The majority (78%) presented 2 to 4 symptoms. The "post-COVID neurological syndrome" represents a diagnostic challenge for the clinical neurologist because of the multiple manifestations: central and peripheral nervous system, musculoskeletal and neuropsychiatric symptoms, without a classical semiology, with intense and constant headache, overuse, insomnia, anxiety and unexplained depression in patients with no previous history. The response to classical treatment is variable, as the symptoms can be varied and widespread (similar to a moth bite). We are just beginning to learn about this complex, novel and highly infectious disease 24).

Inoyatova et al. (2021). The following supposed aetiological factors for the development of the disease were established: bad habits 0.5%, transient ischaemic attack (TIA) 5%, dental disease 10%, severe stress 11%, ear, nose and throat disease (ENT) 19%, frequent colds 26%, frequent hypothermia 26%. On the other hand, concomitant diseases in patients with TN due to diseases of the cardiovascular system: diabetes 2%, obesity 23%, thyroid disease 1%, gastrointestinal tract disease 4%, arteriosclerosis 25%, cardiac ischaemia 14%, hypertonic disease 31%. Indeed, the most commonly affected side of the face is the right (60%), and to a lesser extent the left; but simultaneous bilateral pain in TN is rare (1.7%-5%). However, these patients frequently experience paroxysms of unilateral alternating lateral pain. In terms of pain, the maxillary (V2) and mandibular (V3) branches are most commonly involved, although a quarter of cases affect the ophthalmic division (V1). Thus: only V2 (32.5%), V2 and V3 (42.5%) on the right side of the process (53%). By age range, middle-aged and elderly patients suffer more often from TN at 66.7%, with women predominating at 64.8%. Nevertheless, patients of different ages react heterogeneously to the pain syndrome. The clinical picture of TN is determined by lesions in the branches, the most specific symptoms of which are the presence of trigger zones for the development of pain. On the basis of the data obtained, it was shown that the intensity of the pain syndrome can be judged by means of the Beck Depression Scale and the VAS. The Beck Depression Scale in this study does not reflect an objective picture of acute pain syndrome, especially in the comparison group (25).

Kaya and Kaya (2021). A patient developed acute trigeminal neuritis after Pfizer-BioNTech's SARS-CoV-2 vaccine. The patient recovered completely with steroid treatment. Due to findings including typical features and localisation of pain and activation by some actions, the case was considered as trigeminal neuralgia (TN 2021). Pregabalin was administered to control the pain. However, despite 4 weeks of treatment, the pain persisted and his attacks continued. At the same time, the patient was consulted for toothache. Although the dental X-ray was normal, amoxicillin/clavulanic acid (2x1 g daily) was administered. After use of the first dose of antibiotic, he developed angioedema and his general condition worsened. Methylprednisolone 80 mg intravenously was administered in the emergency department. Later, the patient was discharged home with a 7-day tapering course of steroids. With this treatment, all complaints, including facial, jaw and dental pain, recovered. The patient has been doing well and without recurrence at regular follow-ups for 6 months (9).

Lara C. (2021). It is generally caused by compression of vessels on the nerve, but there are exceptions, where this condition does not develop. There are 4-13 cases per 100,000 inhabitants and mainly in women over 50 years of age. Investigations of radicular demyelination of the nerve, according to Moses, Beaver and Kerr; it is manifested by vascular compression of the posterior radicular region, with the presence of irregular degenerative myelin in the course of the trigeminal nerve and by this segmental demyelination, non-synaptic transmissions are revealed, giving rise to triggers. For their treatment, the drugs of choice are: Carbamazepine, lamotrigine, baclofen, gabapentin, pregabalin, botulinum toxin; finally, wait for a better tolerated drug (26).

Maarbjerg and Benoliel (2021). Globally, the new International Classification of Headache Disorders (ICHD) for TN is based on reliable clinical data, imaging and neurophysiological studies. However, there is a lack of safe and effective medications to manage TN, as well as a lack of solid data on neurosurgical options. Similarly, more research is needed on the associated clinical signs (lacrimation and sensory changes), as well as on all aspects of TN (natural history, clinical picture, diagnosis, treatment and prognosis). In conclusion, research should adhere to the ICHD outline for TN; with emphasis on rigorous investigations of surgical alternatives for the different subtypes of TN and improved pharmacotherapy (2).

Mannerak et al. (2021). About 1-2% of TN cases are inherited. Available human studies propose the following genes as possible contributors to the development of TN: CACNA1A, CACNA1H, CACNA1F, KCNK1, TRAK1, SCN9A, SCN8A, SCN3A, SCN10A, SCN5A, NTRK1, GABRG1, MPZ gene, MAOA gene and SLC6A4. Their role in familial TN remains to be addressed. Experimental animal studies suggest an emerging role of genetics in trigeminal pain, although animal models may be more relevant to trigeminal neuropathic pain than TN per se. In sum, this systematic review suggests a more important role of genetic factors in the pathogenesis of TN than previously assumed (7).

Mo et al. (2021). Patients with trigeminal neuralgia (TN) exhibited reductions in cortical indices in the anterior cingulate cortex (ACC), medial cingulate cortex (MCC) and posterior cingulate cortex (PCC) relative to controls. In addition, they had a generalised reduction in subcortical volume that was most evident in the putamen, thalamus, accumbens, pallidum and hippocampus. The brain-wide morphological alterations successfully allow the automated diagnosis of TN with high specificity (TN: 95.35 %; disease controls: 46.51 %). Ultimately, TN is associated with a distinctive whole-brain structural neuroimaging pattern, underlining the value of machine learning as an approach to differentiate between morphological phenotypes, ultimately revealing the full spectrum of this disease and highlighting relevant diagnostic biomarkers (12).

Molina et al. (2021). Although the PCR test was negative, for the 65-year-old patient, the rapid test showed positive IgM and IgG serology for SARS-CoV-2, and an initial analysis showed a slightly elevated D-dimer of 800 ng/ml (upper limit: 500 ng/ml). Due to these findings, the patient was diagnosed with TN secondary to SARS-CoV-2 viral infection. However, the pain resolved with the improvement of COVID-19 specific symptoms. Therefore, the new SARS-CoV-2 coronavirus is a possible aetiology of secondary TN. However, further studies are needed to elucidate the neuropathology of this viral infection (16).

Mortazavi et al. (2021). The report of a 38-year-old man with atypical odontalgia (OA) who, after undergoing 28 root canal restorations and 4 extractions with pain originating in the left premolar region and radiating to the contralateral mandibular region, neck, head and shoulders, was referred to the maxillofacial surgeon and diagnosed as atypical odontalgia and treated with fluoxetine and clonazepam. It makes it clear that dentists should consider the visual analogue scale (VAS) when confronted with odontalgia without a reasonable organic cause and avoid unnecessary dental procedures (11).

Slettebo (2021). Of 102 patients who consulted for facial pain, 38 patients were first referred to a neurologist, 1 patient to a neurosurgeon and 1 patient to an oral surgeon for surgical treatment of the suspected TN. All these 38 patients had been examined by one or more dentists before consulting their neurologist. The other 64 patients were evaluated for routine follow-ups, for post neurosurgical pain, or for other types of facial pain. Furthermore, overdiagnosis of TN occurred in a significant proportion of patients referred for neurosurgical treatment. The main reason was overestimation of MRI findings: at the expense of a careful history and examination. Consequently, misdiagnosis is an important factor against health, as patients
may face unnecessary risks and futile neurosurgery, in addition to delayed treatment of their underlying painful condition (27).

Smith et al. (2021). The researchers found multiple genetic and molecular targets involved in possible pathophysiologies related to the creation of trigeminal neuralgia. Without a clear candidate genesis, which demonstrates the possibility that the genetic predisposition to trigeminal neuralgia may involve multiple genes and/or downstream products, such as ion channels, therefore, TN could be multi-causal. Thus, the inability of the neurovascular compression model to satisfactorily account for a significant subset of patients with sporadic and familial TN has led to the investigation of alternative models, especially those involving ion channels (6).

Abril et al. (2022). Of 21 articles selected, only 9 were filtered out, of which 3 were case reports and 6 descriptive studies. All of them intercept that the absence of information on TN leads to unnecessary root canal treatment. Therefore, by developing a correct clinical history with adequate complementary examinations, a correct diagnosis can be made and a lack of information on TN can be foreseen, preventing dentists and endodontists from treating root canals without any basis. Therefore, the mastery and information of this pathophysiology would be of particular help to stomatologists and endodontists. Likewise, neurologists and neurosurgeons could differentiate between typical and atypical TN from odontogenic pain (28).

Chen et al. (2022). The aetiology of TN is probably multifactorial in many patients. Only a small percentage of TN patients present with demonstrable compression or morphological changes in the trigeminal nerve, and neurovascular compression does not always translate into disease. In addition, most patients present with a normal physical and neurological examination and reliable biomarkers for the disease are lacking. Therefore, such a complex disease presentation makes accurate diagnosis of

TN difficult; fortunately, surgical and minimally invasive interventions seem to have a promising solution (29).

Jay and Barkin (2022). To be clear, in facial pain; migraine and trigeminal autonomic cephalalgias are localised around the ocular and frontal regions. Although, isolated oral and facial pain with neurovascular features suggestive of facial or orofacial migrania have been reported. In any case, isolated "facial migrania" is very rare (0.2%). It causes misdiagnosis with dental and maxillary sinus pathology. Despite this, TN is often misdiagnosed because of its initial presentation in a primary care setting, with at least three subtypes, whose treatment may be multifactorial. In turn, the diagnostic criteria for TN in The International Classification of Headache Disorders, Edition 3 (ICHD- 3), suggests: recurrent paroxysms of unilateral facial pain in the distribution of one or more divisions of the trigeminal nerve, lasting a fraction of a second to two minutes, severe and electric shock-like, stabbing, or sharp stabbing and may be precipitated by innocuous stimuli both with and without the affected trigeminal dermatome. Therefore, a thorough history and neurological examination are essential to achieve the correct diagnosis (4).

2.3 Theoretical basis

2.3.1 Trigeminal neuralgia (TN)

The trigeminal nerve, a component of two sensory and motor elements, is a large cranial nerve; it starts from the anterior aspect of the pons in two motor and sensory fibres; it runs forward until it reaches the upper portion of the vertex of the petrous section of the temporal bone, within the middle cranial fossa; from it the sensory portion generates the trigeminal ganglion of Gasser, giving rise to the ophthalmic branch (V1) of sensory fibres, with branches: frontal, lacrimal and nasal; upper maxillary (V2) of sensory fibres, with branches: ophthalmic (V1) of sensory fibres, with branches: frontal, lacrimal and nasal: frontal, lacrimal and nasal; maxillary (V2) of sensory fibres, with branches: orbital, sphenopalatine, pterygopalatine, posterior/superior nasal, nasopalatine, palatine and upper dentary; and mandibular (V3) of motor and sensory fibres, with branches: recurrent menmgeo, deep medial temporal, temporomaseterine, temporobuccal, auriculotemporal, inferior dentary, lesser hypoglossal or lingual and mentonian branch (14).

TN or tic doloreux is a very painful disease, which, in order to avoid confusion, headaches or other conditions should be ruled out; moreover, it is currently being supported by imaging (17). It has a prevalence of 4-13 cases per 100,000 inhabitants (18). It is commonly triggered by chewing and manipulation of the gums. Therefore, patients are likely to consult their dentist when it first occurs before being referred to a neurologist or neurosurgeon (3). Notably, TN, with the exception of multiple sclerosis, unilaterally involves the facial area (19). It is rare for TN to present as trigeminal status or rapid succession of tic-like spasms, triggered by any stimulus.

According to their topography, branches V2 and V3 are more affected, as follows: V1 (4%); V2 (23%); V3 (15%); V1 and V2 (16.5%); V2 and V3 (32%) (22). Another example, with locality, facial sinus in 72%, with severe unilateral pain in the V2 branch at the Valleix examination and 47% of cases (22). For another author, the most affected side of the face is the right (60%), and to a lesser extent the left; but simultaneous bilateral pain in TN is rare (1.7%-5%). However, these patients frequently experience paroxysms of unilateral alternating lateral pain. In terms of pain, the maxillary (V2) and mandibular (V3) branches are most commonly involved, although a quarter of cases affect the ophthalmic division (V1). Thus: V2 alone 32.5%, V2 and V3 42.5%; on the right side of the process 53% (25). Other scientific research shows that the right hemiarch is generally affected in 60% of cases, 39% on the left side and 1% bilaterally with alternating pain occurring mainly in cases of multiple sclerosis, which is why 18% of patients with bilateral TN have this pathology. Likewise, the V2 and V3 branches are the most severely damaged branches (42% of cases), the V2 branch alone (20%), the V3 branch alone (17%), V1 and V2 together (14%), and V1, V2 and V3 (5%) and V1 alone (2%) (5). Namely, another investigation also pointed to the right side as the most affected 59.5% in its V2 branch at 33.23% (14). From another angle, in a study 68.9 % showed involvement of the right facial side, where the most affected branch was the mandibular 47.9 % (13).affected was the mandibular branch 47.5% (8). In a survey, the development of TN as a result of a chronic dental infection in this tooth was shown in a 49 year old female patient with a decade of acute, dull, constant pain from mechanical and sensory stimuli located in the V3 branch (20).

Figure 1 *Pain caused by Trigeminal Neuralgia*

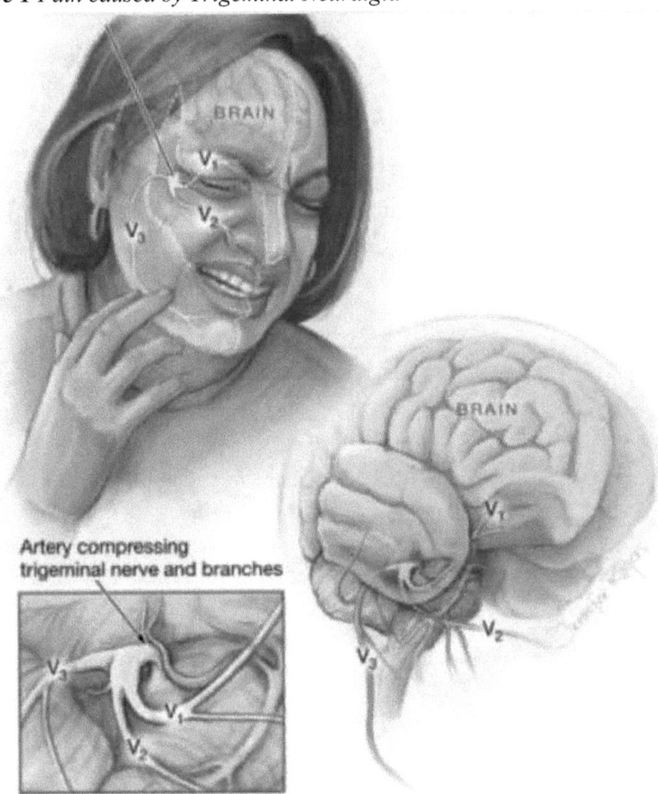

Note: Adapted from Lara (2021).

A good systematic C.H. with adequate anamnesis, detailed dental, periodontal and intraoral examination and a general orofacial radiograph are necessary. Finally, if the case warrants it, further examination techniques are necessary (21). In addition, a thorough history and neurological examination are essential to achieve the correct diagnosis (4). When examining a patient with TN, facial sensitivity, extrinsic ocular musculature, masticatory function of the masseters and pterygoids with the mouth open, with the chin deviating to the diseased side in paresis, should be examined. Finally, the differential diagnosis of TN should take into account herpes zoster with continuous non-paroxysmal pain with vesicles and crusts immediately after the pain distributed in the V1 branch, and in cases of herpes zoster without vesicles, the differential diagnosis becomes complicated; odontalgia; orbital pathology; temporal arteritis with hypersensitivity of the superficial temporal artery and intracranial tumours (5).

As a result of misdiagnosis and undertreatment, there is an urgent need to improve neurological knowledge in order to recognise the clinical picture of TN in a timely manner and to adhere properly to specific guidelines. This may benefit patients whose quality of life is severely affected (1). Likewise, it remains an unknown pathological entity, even poorly managed by specialists (25).

Therefore, disease targeting is an important factor, as patients avoid unnecessary risks such as futile neurosurgery and delayed treatment of their underlying painful condition (27). Since most patients present with a normal physical and neurological examination, there is a lack of reliable biomarkers for the disease (29); therefore, an investigation into all aspects of TN (natural history, clinical picture, diagnosis, treatment and prognosis) is essential (2). Hence, differential diagnoses include odontogenic pain syndromes, as well as atypical orofacial pain; in that sense, the current literature acknowledges the difficulties in correctly diagnosing trigeminal neuralgia, but seems to underestimate the extent (3).

In turn, the diagnostic criteria for TN in The International Classification of Headache Disorders, Edition 3 (ICHD-3), suggest: recurrent paroxysms of unilateral facial pain in the distribution of one or more divisions of the trigeminal nerve, lasting a fraction of a second to two minutes, severe and similar to electric shock, stabbing, or sharp stabbing and may be precipitated by innocuous stimuli both with and without the affected trigeminal dermatome (4). On the other hand, the American Academy of Neurology (AAN), developed a new taxonomy with diagnostic accuracy criteria, with a classification system for neuropathic pain, created to be applied in diagnostic and treatment decisions (19). In this way, when faced with situations of TN with atypical clinical features, it is essential to carry out a cranial MRI, which is fundamental for any TN (5).

Furthermore, brain-wide morphological alterations successfully allow automated diagnosis of TN with high specificity (TN: 95.35 %; disease controls: 46.51 %). Ultimately, TN is associated with a distinctive whole-brain structural neuroimaging pattern, underlining the value of machine learning as an approach to differentiate between morphological phenotypes, ultimately revealing the full spectrum of this disease and highlighting relevant diagnostic biomarkers (12).

One can cite this article in which the final diagnosis was made by a neurologist or headache specialist 85.3%, and the mean interval between onset of the disease and diagnosis by a specialist was 10.8 ± 21.2 months. The "diagnostic delay" was 7.2 ± 12.5 months and diagnostic errors were found at the first consultation in 42.1% of cases. Instrumental and laboratory investigations were performed in 93.1% of the patients before the final diagnosis of TN. The misdiagnoses were: dental problems 37.48 %, including odontalgia, periodontal abscess, caries, dental granulomas; sinusitis 14.3%; unspecified facial pain 9.1%; unspecified headache 7.8%; migraine 6.5%; cluster headache 5.2%; temporomandibular joint dysfunction 3.9%; glaucoma tension headache 1.3%, otitis 1.3%; tonsillitis 1.3% (1).

In the therapeutic field, mainly to prevent dentists and endodontists from unfounded root canal treatment (28) (5). As such, other researchers conclude that it is not uncommon for patients to be passed from one specialist to another, even to dentists, and sometimes undergo unnecessary and ineffective dental treatments such as root canals and extractions, contributing to their daily ailment (23).

Illustrating the casuistry, a 73 year old patient underwent root canal treatment in 22, 23, 25 and the latter with apicoectomy, in addition to root canals in 24 and 26, when the actual diagnosis was TN type I (13). Similarly, in another investigation, it was evaluated whether patients underwent root canal treatment for undiagnosed TN; out of 187 patients, 117 participated. About 55.5% of the patients had odontalgia and 65.8% visited the dentist. About 41.8% of patients underwent a dental procedure; 18.8% had worsening pain, while 8.5% had some partial improvement. About 19.6% also underwent root canal treatment, while 6.8% had a nerve block.

Namely, this other case report describes the application of major autohaemotherapy, 3 sessions for 14 days prior to the exodontia of the 36th tooth to facilitate the resolution of TN, without any symptomatology at the 4-month follow-up (20).

One investigation highlights that, carbamazepine was the most prescribed drug with a median dose of 600 mg (RIQ: 400 - 1000 mg). Two thirds of patients reported prominent satisfaction. The mean (± SD) dose of carbamazepine used to control pain was significantly higher among those with a history of tooth extraction compared to those without a history of tooth extraction. A statistically significant number of patients with single-branch involvement reported outstanding satisfaction with their treatment compared with those with more than one branch involvement (8). Well, intravenous phenytoin is very effective; however, individuals with typical TN improve with carbamazepine initially, which is rare in atypical facial pain (5). In conclusion, a current review proposes the following drugs in order of choice: carbamazepine, lamotrigine, baclofen, gabapentin, pregabalin, botulinum toxin; finally, waiting for a better tolerated drug (26).

Ultimately, there is a need for a better understanding of the disease among dentists and patients for timely and correct treatment, without resorting to exodontia. For this reason, the onus is on neurosurgeons/neurologists to disseminate knowledge about proper diagnosis and treatment modalities (10). If not treated properly, it can lead to stress at work, social, psychological and even suicide (17).

In short, it can be divided into primary, idiopathic or essential and secondary or symptomatic (5).

Figure 2 *Facial and intraoral innervation of the trigeminal nerve (white areas due to cervical nerves, light grey areas intrabuccally on tongue and throat due to glossopharyngeal nerves).*

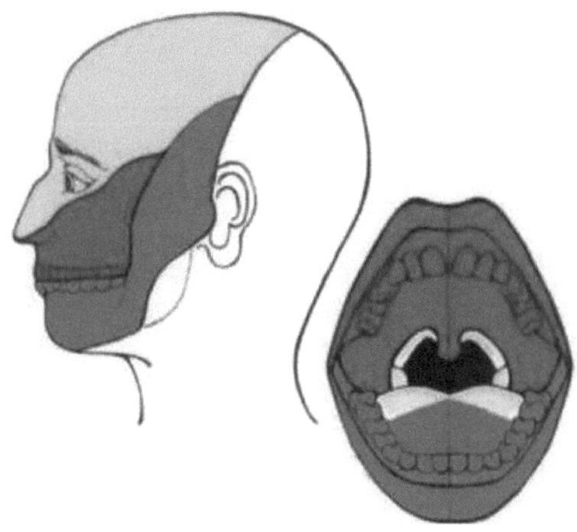

Note: Adapted from Alcantara and Montero (2017).

2.3.1.1Primary or classical. These are the most common and it is not possible to know the

stimulus that provokes it (5). By vascular compression, it is necessary to demonstrate morphological changes in the trigeminal nerve root (19). Whereas, in a clinical study, 90.2% of patients met criteria for classic TN, in addition, 9.8% had symptomatic TN (8).

2.3.1.2 Secondary or symptomatic. There is an underlying cause, clinically presenting paresthesia and dysesthesia, where the pain becomes a secondary condition with deficient signs on neurological examination. It is very common to present a picture of atypical neuralgia and in its onset, it is sometimes confused with primary neuralgia; its causes are due to lesions of the pontocerebellar angle, damaging the brain stem, different diseases of Meckel's cavum, tumours of the middle fossa, metastasis of the base of the skull, pituitary adenomas, etc. Another lesion causing TN with very similar features to the essential lesion is multiple sclerosis, which presents a neuralgia of this type (5). Another study, coincidentally, highlights the underlying neurological disease or tumour of the pontocerebellar angle (19).

2.3.1.3 Idiopathic or essential. It is so called because it is unknown (19); therefore, mastery and information on this pathophysiology would help stomatologists. From another perspective, neurologists and neurosurgeons could differentiate typical and atypical TN from odontogenic pain (28,5).

Also, not to confuse odontogenic pain with non-odontogenic pain (myofascial, trigeminal neuropathy, as well as painful post-traumatic trigeminal neuropathic pain, orofacial neurovascular pain, cardiac and paranasal sinus disease) (21).

2.3.1.4Pain . Occurs when eating, brushing the teeth, etc.

The symptoms of TN are determined clinically by lesions in the branches, the most specific symptoms of which are the presence of trigger zones for the development of pain, in which the intensity of the pain syndrome can be judged by means of the Beck

depression scale and the VAS (25).
The report of a study on a case of atypical odontalgia (AO) in a 38 year old man who, after undergoing 28 root canal restorations and 4 extractions with pain originating in the left premolar region and radiating to the contralateral mandibular region, neck, head and shoulders, was referred to the maxillofacial surgeon diagnosed as atypical odontalgia and treated with fluoxetine and clonazepam. It makes it clear that dentists should consider the "visual analogue scale (VAS)" when confronted with pulpitis without a reasonable organic cause and avoid unnecessary dental procedures (11).
Neuralgia is generated as a consequence of a trauma or variation of some afferent structures of the peripheral nervous system, according to "The international Association for the study of pain", it is a pain of varying degrees of intensity, which travels along the route of the nerve or nerve root, representing a type of peripheral neuropathic style algia and generally unilateral (14). Other research also highlights an abrupt, spontaneous onset lasting from a few seconds to two minutes, with paroxysms triggered by harmless mechanical stimuli or movements, but if, in addition, they experience additional continuous pain, then they manifest TN with continuous pain (19).
To illustrate, in one scientific study, most participants reported mixed types of pain, such as burning, shooting and electric shock-like; a well-defined trigger zone was identified in one third (36 %) of cases (8).
According to one study report, 86% of patients consulted a physician at the first attacks of pain. The specialists consulted before diagnosis of TN were: primary care physicians (PCP) 43.1%, dentists 30.4%, otolaryngologists 3.9%, neurosurgeons 3.9%, neurologists or headache specialists 14.7%, others 8% (1). In a separate case, 102 patients came to the clinic for facial pain, with 38 patients being referred for the first time to a neurologist, 1 patient to a neurosurgeon and 1 patient to an oral surgeon for surgical treatment of the suspected TN; and all 38 patients had previously been examined by one or more dentists before consulting their neurologist (27).

***Table 1** Differential diagnostics to consider*

Affection of the trigeminal nerve	-Tumours -Multiple sclerosis plates -Herpes Zoster
Trigeminal deafferentation pain syndrome	**-Atypical orofacial pain, Neuropathic trigeminal pain**
Dental Disease	**-Musculo-facial y joint disease -Joint disease temporomandibular**
Vascular disease	**-Temporal arthritis -Migranas**
Other	**-Other types of headache -Referred pain of orbits and sinuses -Psychogenic causes**

Note: Adapted from Lara (2021).

2.3.2 Most common aetiology

The following supposed aetiological factors for the development of the disease were established: bad habits 0.5%, transient ischaemic attack (TIA) 5%, dental disease 10%, severe stress 11%, ear, nose and throat disease (ENT) 19%, frequent colds 26%, frequent hypothermia 26% (25). On the other hand, concomitant diseases in patients with TN due to diseases of the cardiovascular system: diabetes 2%, obesity 23%, thyroid disease 1%, gastrointestinal tract disease 4%, arteriosclerosis 25%, cardiac ischaemia 14%, hypertonic disease 31% (25).

2.3.2.1 Predisposing factors

Age. In particular, the age range between 50-90 years is presented (22); another study also highlights that it occurs over 50 years around 63 years of age (5). Similarly, another study highlights that this condition is greater in patients over 50 years of age and especially in those diagnosed with multiple sclerosis with an incidence of 1 to 2%, impacting the ability to work in 34% of patients (18). It should not be forgotten that this pathology presents as odontogenic pain, so it is urgent that stomatologists are aware of its symptoms (13). Finally, by age range, middle-aged and elderly patients suffer more often from TN at 66.7%, although patients of different ages react heterogeneously to the pain syndrome (25). Another investigation claims that the pain picture appeared in a young patient; remembering that typical TN is frequent in patients over 50 years of age (5).

Gender. In short, it is more common in females, as they are the most affected (76.7%) (14, 17). Similarly, one study found that, according to gender, 67% are female and 33% male (20). Another study puts the female predominance at 64.8% (25); thus, a recent study indicates that the majority of the audience is female, aged 50 and over (26). On the contrary, according to some authors it is more frequent in men (1.2:1) and for others it is more frequent in women (5). In a report on atypical odontalgia (OA) of dull, chronic, constant pain; prevalent in women between 53 and 62 years of age, with an average duration of 24 months; especially in depressed, anxious patients, with somatic pain, insomnia, obsessive-compulsive, eating and personality disorders. Another trigger may be after dental care, endodontics, exodontics and prostheses (11).

2.3.2.2 Aetiological factors

COVID. The "post-COVID neurological syndrome" represents a diagnostic challenge for the neurological clinician because of the multiple manifestations: central and peripheral nervous system, musculoskeletal and neuropsychiatric symptoms, without a classical semiology, with intense and constant headache, overuse, insomnia, anxiety and unexplained depression in patients with no previous history (24).

It is understood that, the new SARS-CoV-2 coronavirus is a possible aetiology of secondary TN. However, further studies are needed to elucidate the neuropathology of this viral infection (16). Thus, for example in one investigation, a patient despite 4 weeks of treatment, the pain persisted and her attacks continued. At the same time, the patient was consulted for odontalgia. Although the dental X-ray was normal, amoxicillin/clavulanic acid (2x1 g daily) was administered. After use of the first dose of antibiotic, he developed angioedema and his general condition worsened. Methylprednisolone 80 mg intravenously was administered in the emergency department and she was discharged, because she had actually developed acute trigeminal neuritis after the Pfizer-BioNTech vaccine against SARS-CoV-2 (9).

Genetics. The researchers found multiple genetic and molecular targets involved in possible pathophysiologies that are related to the development of trigeminal neuralgia. It has been shown that, genetic predisposition to trigeminal neuralgia may involve multiple genes and/or downstream products, such as ion channels, thus TN may be multi-causal (6). About 1-2% of TN cases have a hereditary form. Available human studies propose the following genes as possible contributors to the development of TN: CACNA1A, CACNA1H, CACNA1F, KCNK1, TRAK1, SCN9A, SCN8A, SCN3A, SCN10A, SCN5A, NTRK1, GABRG1, MPZ gene, MAOA gene and SLC6A4. Thus, there is a more important role of genetic factors in the pathogenesis of TN than previously assumed (7). The annual incidence is 4 cases per 100,000 inhabitants and for this researcher it is rarely genetic (5); similar to a Spanish study, with an incidence of 4 to 13 people per 100,000 inhabitants (26).

Tumour. Within TN, the symptomatic mode secondary to skull base tumours, multiple sclerosis and compressive vascular anomalies is common. The aetiology of this neuropathic type of pain remains unknown, although the pathophysiological mechanism is thought to be compression of the trigeminal nerve by blood vessels such as cerebral arteries in the access zone of the root of the pons (14). In cases where TN is the effect of a brain tumour, it has atypical features of constant pain, with deficient signs on neurological examination with loss of sensation; sometimes the examination is initially normal in some patients. If, on examination of a non-operated patient, a neurological deficit is found, a structural cause of the neuralgia should be considered, e.g. tumour, multiple sclerosis, etc. (5). However, acoustic neurinoma is the most common. On the other hand, tumours of the posterior fossa are the most common causes of neuralgia that appear to be typical or true (5).

The association of brain tumour and TN is less than 0.8%, particularly as a brain tumour within TN, where facial pain may occur contralateral to the tumour lesion, due to slippage caused by the mass in the brainstem (5).

Figure 3 *New systematic approach to classification and diagnosis of TN*

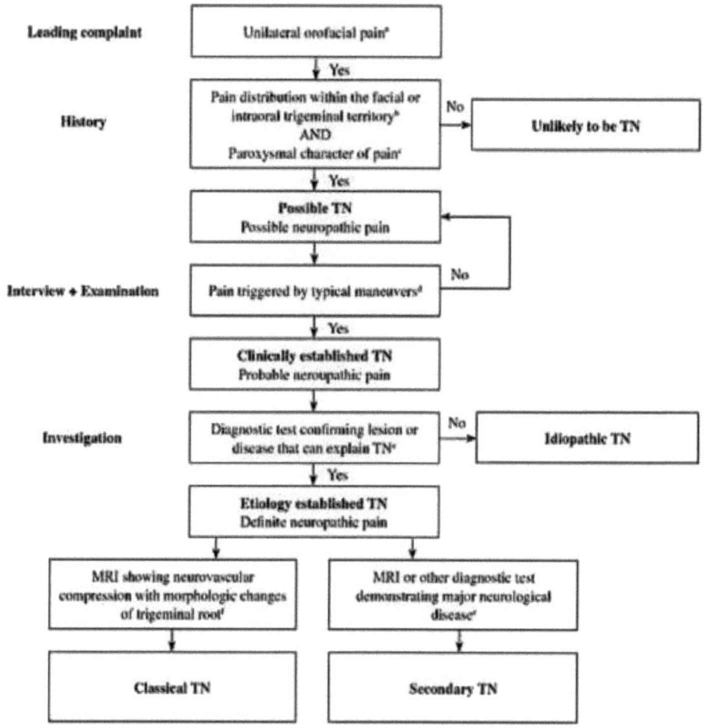

Leading complaint — Unilateral orofacial pain[a]

Yes ↓

History — Pain distribution within the facial or intraoral trigeminal territory[b] AND Paroxysmal character of pain[c] — No → **Unlikely to be TN**

Yes ↓

Possible TN
Possible neuropathic pain

↓

Interview + Examination — Pain triggered by typical maneuvers[d] — No → (back to Possible TN)

Yes ↓

Clinically established TN
Probable neuropathic pain

↓

Investigation — Diagnostic test confirming lesion or disease that can explain TN[e] — No → **Idiopathic TN**

Yes ↓

Etiology established TN
Definite neuropathic pain

↓ MRI showing neurovascular compression with morphologic changes of trigeminal root[f] → **Classical TN**

↓ MRI or other diagnostic test demonstrating major neurological disease[e] → **Secondary TN**

Note: Adapted from Alcantara and Montero (2017).

Demyelination Investigations of the radicular demyelination of the nerve, according to Moses, Beaver and Kerr; it is manifested by vascular compression of the posterior radicular region, with the presence of irregular degenerative myelin in the course of the trigeminal nerve and by this segmental demyelination, non-synaptic transmissions are revealed, giving rise to triggers (26).

Biologically, it is caused by specific abnormalities of the trigeminal afferent neurons, either in the trigeminal root or trigeminal ganglion, causing the axons to be hyper-excitable with paroxysmal pain discharges. Such post-discharge bursts can be triggered by an external stimulus and prolonged beyond the duration of the stimulus; or recruit neighbouring neurons triggering an electrical action with paroxysmal pain by close contact between the fibres (14).

Unknown aetiology Usually due to compression of vessels on the nerve, but there are exceptions, where this condition does not develop (26), or according to Girija (pp. 23-29), the cause is not known (30).

2.4 Glossary of terms

Trigeminal nerve, trigeminal neuralgia, pain, etiology, age, gender, COVID, genetics, tumour, neurology, neurosurgery, dentistry.

CHAPTER 3

METHODOLOGY

3.1 Operationalisation of the variables

Operationalised in this way:

Variable X: Most common aetiology

Variable Y: Trigeminal neuralgia

3.1.1 Variable X: Most Common Aetiology

Conceptual definition. Reductions in cortical indices in the anterior, medial and posterior cingulate cortex, as well as subcortical volume in putamen, thalamus, accumbens, pallidum and hippocampus (12).

Dimensions: The following are considered:

Predisposing factors:

- Age
- Sex
- Ano

Aetiological factors:

- COVID
- Genetics
- Tumour Cause
- Demyelination
- Etiology unknown

3.1.2 Variable Y: Trigeminal neuralgia

Conceptual definition. It is a painful condition of a particular severity or neuropathic pain (23).

Dimensions: The following are considered:

Classical

Secondary

Idiopathic

Pain

3.1.3. Operationalisation of variables

The operationalisation is presented in the following tables: Perez (2019)

***Table 2** Operationalization of variable X*

Variable Independent	Definition Conceptual	Definition Operational	Dimensions	Indicators	Measurement scale	Index	Instrument
Most common aetiology	In this regard, Mo et al. (2021) found reductions in cortical indices in the anterior, medial and posterior cingulate cortex, as well as reductions in subcortical volume in the putamen, thalamus, accumbens, pallidum and hippocampus (12).	Variable measured by means of medical records collected for this study from the areas of neurology, neurosurgery and dentistry.	*Predisposing factors* Age Sex *Ano* *Etiological factors* - COVID - Demyelination - Unknown aetiology	*- 20-40* *- 41-60* *- 61-80* *- 81-99* *-Male -Female* *2019* *2020* *2021* *2022* *- Yes - No - Not recorded - Test positive - Test negative - Vaccinated - Not vaccinated* *- Yes -No -Not recorded - White ethnicity -Mestizo ethnicity - Indigenous ethnicity -Afro-descendant ethnicity* *Yes No No registration* *- Yes* *- With MRI - No - Without MRI - No record - NR MRI* *Yes No No registration*	*Ordinal* *Nominal* *Ordinal* *Nominal* *Nominal* *Nominal* *Nominal* *Nominal*	*Always 1* *Frequent 2* *Sometimes 3* *Never 4*	*-Quantitative observation - Recording tables -Clinical records*

Genelica
Tumour Cause

Variable Dependent	Definition Conceptual	Definition Operational	Dimensions	Indicators	Scale of measurement	Index	Instrument
Trigeminal neuralgia	In this respect, Bara et al. (2021), a painful condition of a particular severity o neuropathic pain (23).	Variable measured by means of medical records collected for this study from the areas of neurology, neurosurgery and dentistry. Integrating knowledge	Classical Secondary Idiopathic Not registered (19) Pain (25, 19)	-Morphological changes in the trigeminal nerve root due to vascular compression. -For identifiable underlying neurological disease (portocerebellar angle tumour, multiple sclerosis). - Of unknown aetiology. - *Visual analogue scale (VAS).* Horizontal line of 10 centimetres, at the ends of which are the opposite expressions of pain. To the left is the absence or lesser intensity and to the right the greater intensity (11). *-Mentally handicapped,* through gestures and/or body language y other criteria	Nominal Ordinal Nominal	Always 1 Frequent 2 Sometimes 3 Never 4 Painless/NR (0) Mild pain (1-3) Moderate pain (4-6) Severe pain (7-10) Grimaces (yes/no/NR) Pupillary dilatation (yes/no/NR) Referred to Lima (yes/no/NR) Frequency (Daily/Weekly/NR)	-Quantitative observation -Registration tables -Clinical case histories
				-Pain test Alcántara and González (19).	Ordinal Nominal	-Affected branches: *V1, V2,V3, V1/V2, V2/V3, V1/V2/V3, V1/V2/V3, NR* -Affected side: *Right/* Left/ *Right/ Left/ Left* Both, NR -Onset of pain: Mild/Moderate/Moderate / *Brusco, NR* Duration: 1 *second to 2* minutes/ -Duration: 1	

	second to 2 minutes More than 2 minutes, NR -Type of pain: *provoked/ Spontaneous/ NR* Stimulus elicited: None/ *Mechanically safe/ Movements/ NR* -Pain between paroxysms: (Yes)/ *(No)/ (No) (NR)* -Continuous additional pain: (Yes)/*(No)/ (NR)*

Pain test Alcantara y Gonzalez (19).

3.2 Type and design of research

Type of research

It is non-experimental, qualitative, quantitative, retrospective and cross-sectional.

Study design:

It corresponds to descriptive correlational research. Ballester (2004) states that "it is oriented towards determining the degree of relationship existing between two or more variables of interest in the same sample of subjects or the degree of relationship between two observed phenomena or events" (p.79). It leads us to understand the degree of dependence between them, where what happens in one variable triggers changes in the other(s)" they continue (31).

Its outline being:

Figure 4 *Outline of the research design*

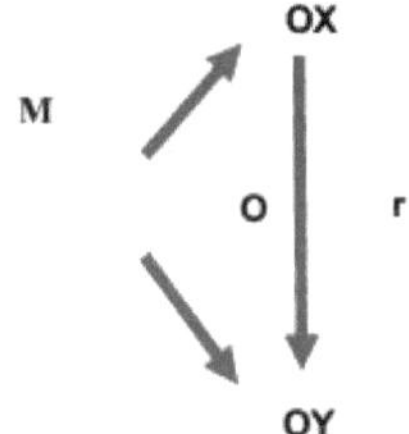

In this way:

M= Study sample

Sub-indices OX= (most common aetiology) and OY (trigeminal neuralgia).

O= checks per variable r= variable ratios established.

The descriptive method exists; in this respect, Perez (2019) "consists of specifying, analysing and systematically interpreting a set of facts related to other variables as they occur in the present" (p.79) (15). In fact, Gallardo (1999) and Ballester (2004), are concerned with providing explanations of the nature under study, therefore, there is no alteration in the variables analysed (32,31).

3.3 Population and Sample

3.3.1. Population

The population, 255 clinical records containing a diagnosis of trigeminal neuralgia in the areas of Neurology, Neurosurgery and Dentistry of the Adolfo Guevara Velasco Hospital from 2019 to August 2022.

3.3.2. Sample

It was obtained in a non-probabilistic manner, consisting of 127 clinical records that met the inclusion criteria with a diagnosis of trigeminal neuralgia from the areas of Neurology, Neurosurgery and Dentistry of the Hospital Nacional Adolfo Guevara Velasco in the interval January 2019 to August 2022; the instrument and unit of analysis to be used, the computerised data of the clinical history and the method was indirect observation.

3.4 Data Collection Instruments

Designed through a table of records to evaluate the variables under study: The instruments will be characterised by being formal and structured.

Variable X:

-Quantitative observation

-Registration tables

-Computerised data from medical records

Variable Y:

-Quantitative observation

-Registration tables

- Computerised data from medical records

3.4.1 Selection criteria

Inclusion Criteria:

The following criteria shall be considered for inclusion (14):

- Computerised data of clinical histories from the Neurology, Neurosurgery and Odontology services that indicate trigeminal neuralgia as a diagnosis and that have been diagnosed by doctors from these disciplines at the Adolfo Guevara Velasco National Hospital.
- Computerised data from medical records with diagnoses dating back to January from 2019 to August 2022 at the Adolfo Guevara Velasco National Hospital.
- Patients over 20 years old

Exclusion Criteria:

The following aspects shall be taken into consideration for their exclusion (15):

- Computer data from medical records for which the diagnosis of trigeminal neuralgia is not definitive.
- Computerised data from medical records whose diagnosis does not specify age, gender, affected facial area and injured limb.
- Computerised data of clinical records with diagnoses after August 2022 at the Adolfo Guevara Velasco National Hospital.

3.4.2 Design or procedure

Administrative

By sending a request to the director of the National Hospital Adolfo Guevara Velasco

Dr. Julio Cesar Espinoza Latorre, to have the participation of the areas of Neurology, Neurosurgery and Dentistry in the collection of information based on physical or computer data.

It happened in phases:

First phase; Process in mesa de partes to obtain the consent to see if the research is feasible, filling out all the corresponding annexes with the processing of the research protocol, finally once the research project was presented for approval by the head of the office of training and teaching EsSalud, the corresponding resolution-authorisation was obtained to develop this research.

Second phase; based on similar NT research, found in search engines in Pub Med, SciELO and Google academic, national and international indexed journals, both in English and Spanish; a data collection sheet was carried out, duly reviewed and evaluated by specialists in the area of trigeminal neuralgia in which it was included:

For variable X "Most common aetiology", the following dimensions were taken: Predisposing factors; (age, sex and year) and aetiological factors: (COVID, genetics, tumour, demyelination and unknown aetiology). The categories were: Yes, No and No Record. For the variable Y "Trigeminal neuralgia", the following dimensions were taken: Classical, secondary, idiopathic; in which category the No Record was added (19). While for the pain scales; the *visual analogue scale (VAS)* without pain or NR (0), mild (1-3), moderate (4-6), intense (7-10) (11); *scale for mentally handicapped* and other criteria: Grimaces (yes/no/NR), pupillary dilation (yes/no/NR), referred to Lima (yes/no/NR), frequency of pain (daily/weekly/NR); to conclude, *the Alcantara and Gonzalez pain test:* Affected branches: (V1), (V2), (V3), (V1/V2), (V2/V3), (V1/V2/V3) and NR; affected side: Right/ Left/ Both/NR; onset of pain: Mild/ Moderate/ Abrupt/NR, duration: 1Second to 2 minutes/ Greater than 2 minutes/ NR; type of pain: Provoked/ Spontaneous/NR; provoked stimulus: None/ Innocuous mechanical/ Movements/NR; pain between paroxysms: (Yes)/ (No)/ NR and additional continuous pain: (Yes)/ (No)/ NR (25, 19, 18). Subsequently, the medical data that met the inclusion criteria were selected and the purpose of data collection in the different specialties was explained to each head of area involved in the study.

Third phase; the pilot test was developed, in video conference with the ZOOM application, together with the neurologist involved in this research Dr. Oscar Francisco Gonzales Gamarra, together with my colleague Dr. Iriana Pena Manrique and the endodontic specialist CD. Nicolas Leon Perez, to avoid any kind of bias; finally, a filter with Dr. Victor Edwin Ore Montalvo. Finally, the results of the test and the data collection sheets were evaluated by a neurologist examiner involved in the research.

Fourth phase or definitive test; having obtained the respective permission of the authorities of EsSalud, on the date, place and time agreed, together with the data with diagnoses G50.0 of Trigeminal Neuralgia of the Hospital Adolfo Guevara Velasco, provided in a USB, by the statistician Jaime Yanez Garcia, of the area of Statistics in the Office of Planning, we proceeded to collect the data in a Mac Book Pro 14-inch laptop, using the Microsoft Excel 2022 programme. In the first visit, corresponding to

5 working days, with the permission of the head of the Neurology Unit, Dr. Victor Edwin Ore Montalvo, the data of 255 clinical histories was investigated in computer of all the cases of patients diagnosed with trigeminal neuralgia (TN); all this casuistry managed from January 2019 to August 2022. Already for the second visit, corresponding to another five working days, the same evaluations were carried out, including data from clinical histories in patients with surgical treatment for TN; in the last visit, also corresponding to another five working days, with permission of the head in charge of Dentistry the C.D. Vidal Pedro Soto Santacruz, the dates of all the clinical histories of the patients diagnosed with trigeminal neuralgia were reviewed, especially the dates with massive root canal treatment, multiple exodontia, cases of the same dental piece that had undergone root canal treatment, exodontia on very close dates and those dental prosthetic treatments that were triggers for TN. In order to collect the information in an orderly and bias-free manner, the Excel programme was used, configuring the information contained in the instruments; For the variable X most common aetiology with the dimension (predisposing factors) age, sex, year of admission of the patient to EsSalud Cusco and for pragmatic purposes "national identity document and medical history number" and in the dimension (aetiological factors) COVID, test +, test-, vaccinated against COVID, not vaccinated against COVID, genetics or ethnic family history, tumour cause, demyelination and unknown aetiology. For the variable TN: Types of TN and the pain scales: VAS visual analogue scale; scale for the mentally handicapped and other criteria "grimacing, pupillary dilation, frequency of pain, referred to Lima"; and Alcantara and Gonzales pain test "affected branch, affected side, onset of pain, duration, type of pain, provoked stimulus, pain between paroxysms and additional continuous pain". In such a way that all the information is useful, practical and easy to process for statistical purposes (15).
The fifth phase, the evaluation of the results, was assigned to a single evaluator, using duly calibrated criteria. The numerical data from the data collection were entered into a data table, adding columns and interpreting the scores of the casuistry found; the interpretation was done by determining ranges, where the cut-offs were established by the researcher and the Gold standard in the study. The distribution and analysis of the ability to take information was carried out thanks to the optical control in frequency distribution tables, as well as the figures. Gonzales et al. (2007), the relationship of the score based on the pathogenesis of TN was carried out thanks to Pearson's partial correlation coefficient, and finally the correlation was interpreted according to values suggested by Cohen's Kappa (31).

- Technical characteristics of the instruments and materials; the data collection instruments were formal and structured, of an informative and instructive nature, towards more objective and truthful data (33).
- Calibration of the inspectors and the main examiner who evaluated the different medical and dental data of trigeminal neuralgia took place at the beginning of the study with discussions on the judgement of the different possible genesis of 5th cranial nerve neuralgia, with the neurologists Dr. Gonzales and Dr. Ore serving as referents.

The intraclass correlation coefficient was used to determine the reliability in the course of measurement (33, 32).

- Methods used and decisions taken for the analysis of the information; the results obtained were recorded in files for this purpose, and were examined using the IBM SPSS programme, version 20. The most common aetiology and trigeminal neuralgia variables were examined, with their respective dimensions, and the findings were expressed as percentages (33, 15).

3.4.3 Reliability of instruments

The basic principles of the research were fulfilled through a licence document to review the computerised data of the medical records of the Hospital Nacional Adolfo Guevara Velasco EsSalud- Cusco, in the years 2019 to August 2022; In addition, the ethical evaluation of these medical records was developed in order to collect the required information and data and thus meet the relevant objectives, keeping the confidentiality and anonymity of the data and information collected and based on similar studies, found in search engines both in Pub Med, SciELO and Google academic (14), from national and international indexed journals, both in English and Spanish. The experts who validated the test were specialists in neurology and dentistry (33). From another angle, to quantify the degree of reliability of the instrument to be calibrated, both for the variable (X): most common aetiology, and for the variable (Y) trigeminal neuralgia, the Cronbach's alpha test was used, whose value was a high reliability of .739 (15,33):

***Table 4** Reliability statistics*

Reliability statistics		
Cronbach's alpha	Cronbach's alpha based on standardised items	N of elements
.739	.773	13

***Table 5** Elemental ladlslics*

Element statistics			
Mean Dev.	DeviationN		
VAR00001	1.09	.378	127
VAR00002	1.06	.302	127
VAR00003	1.03	.250	127
VAR00004	1.02	.125	127
VAR00005	1.31	.675	127
VAR00006	1.38	.745	127
VAR00007	1.93	.669	127
VAR00008	1.08	.390	127
VAR00009	1.08	.390	127
VAR00010	1.44	.626	127
VAR00011	2.56	.832	127
VAR00012	1.83	.949	127
VAR00013	2.17	.952	127

***Table 6** Correlation matrix between elements*

Matrix of correlations between elements

	VA R1	VA R2	VA R3	VA R4	VA R5	VA R6	VA R7	VA R8	VA R9	VA R 10	VA RR 11	VA 12	VA R 13
VA	1.00										-		

VAR1	1.000	.716	.306	.306	.017	-.061	.119	.061	.061	.039	-.029	.040	.024
VAR2	.716	1.000	.604	.604	.135	-.036	.219	.092	.092	-.022	-.015	.009	.127
VAR3	.306	.604	1.000	1.000	.223	.106	.203	.300	.300	.113	.067	.089	.110
VAR4	.306	.604	1.000	1.000	.223	.106	.203	.300	.300	.113	.067	.089	.110
VAR5	.017	.135	.223	.223	1.000	.124	.261	.026	.026	.176	.193	.206	.285
VAR6	-.061	-.036	.106	.106	.124	1.000	.166	.006	.006	-.037	.194	.067	.052
VAR7	.119	.219	.203	.203	.261	.166	1.000	.143	.143	.379	.428	.506	.605
VAR8	.061	.092	.300	.300	.026	.006	.143	1.000	1.000	.247	.010	.164	.134
VAR9	.061	.092	.300	.300	.026	.006	.143	1.000	1.000	.247	.010	.164	.134
VAR10	.039	-.022	.113	.113	.176	-.037	.379	.247	.247	1.000	.224	.525	.470
VAR11	-.029	-.015	.067	.067	.193	.194	.428	.010	.010	.224	1.000	.329	.478
VAR12	.040	.009	.089	.089	.206	.067	.506	.164	.164	.525	.329	1.000	.656
VAR13	.024	.127	.110	.110	.285	.052	.605	.134	.134	.470	.478	.656	1.000

***Table** 7 Statistics of total elements*

	Statistics of total elements				
	Scale average if the element has been removed	Scale variance if the element has been suppressed	Total correlation of elements corrected	Multiple squared correlation	Cronbach's alpha if the item has been removed
VAR00001	17.90	15.108	.125		..743
VAR00002	17.92	14.994	.228		..736
VAR00003	17.95	14.887	.347		..732
VAR00004	17.97	15.237	.375		..736
VAR00005	17.67	13.604	.313		..729
VAR00006	17.61	14.383	.121		..756
VAR00007	17.06	12.164	.645		..686
VAR00008	17.91	14.594	.292		..731
VAR00009	17.91	14.594	.292		..731
VAR00010	17.54	13.075	.476		..709
VAR00011	16.43	12.453	.421		..717
VAR00012	17.15	11.049	.581		..690
VAR00013	16.81	10.631	.658		..674

3.4.4 Ethical aspects

Informed consent

As indicated in Annex 4.

Data confidentiality

Strategies for managing the confidentiality of identifiable data, storage controls, manipulation and personal data sharing in this research proposal followed the following requirements: The necessary data were collected, without using personally identifiable information, and withdrawn immediately after data collection. On the other hand, no unencrypted personal data were leaked for any reason. Furthermore, no original collection documents, in this case computerised, were retained once they had been validated and transferred to an analysis package.

3.5 Validation of the instruments

The experts who validated the test were specialists involved in trigeminal neuralgia (neurologists, neurosurgeons and dentists).

***Table 8** Expert validation*

N.°	EXPERTS	VARIABLE X	VARIABLE Y
1	Dr. Ore	100%	
2	C.D. Soto	100%	
3	Dr. Gonzales		100%
Total		100%	100%

According to expert judgement, a value for both X= 100% and Y= 100% was achieved; to show high applicability of the sample under study.

3.6 Execution budget

There was no external funding or sponsorship for this research.

CHAPTER 4

RESULTS AND DISCUSSION

4.1 Analysis, interpretation and discussion of results ***4.1.1 Descriptive statistics.***

In order to identify the most common aetiology of trigeminal neuralgia in patients treated in EsSalud Cusco from January 2019 to August 2022, 255 patients were reviewed, taking as a sample 127 medical records from the Neurology, Neurosurgery and Dentistry services that indicated trigeminal neuralgia as a diagnosis between January 2019 and August 2022 and in the Adolfo Guevara Velasco National Hospital.

4.1.1.1 Results for the Most Common Aetiology Variable

- Dimension Predisposing Factors

i. **Age**

Table 9 *Age frequency table*

	Frequency	Percentage	Valid percentage	Cumulative percentage	
20 a 40 years	16	12,6	12,6	12,6	
41 to 60 years	53	41,7	41,7	54,3	
Valid					
61 to 80 years	53	41,7	41,7	96,1	
81 to 95 years		53,9		3,9	100,0
Total	127	100,0	100,0		

Figure 5 Age

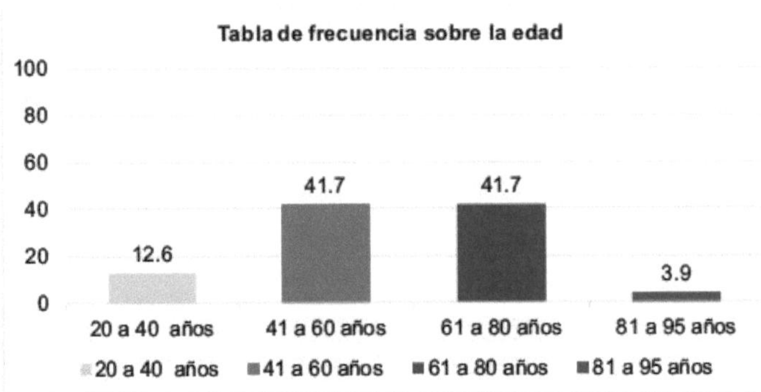

Source: SPSS Vs26

Interpretation and analysis: Table 1 shows the distribution of the population according to age; it is made up of 16 people between 20 and 40 years of age, which is equivalent to 12.In the same way, 53 people were between 41 and 60 years of age (41.7%), 53 people were between 61 and 80 years of age (41.7%), and 5 people were between 81 and 95 years of age (3.9%) of the patients who presented with Trigeminal Neuralgia, which is consistent with the literature.

ii. **Sex**

Table 10 *Sex frequency table*

	Frequency	Percentage	Valid percentage	Cumulative percentage
Female	100	79,5	79,5	79,5
Valid				
Male		2720,5	20,6	100,0
Total	127	100,0		

Figure 6 Gender

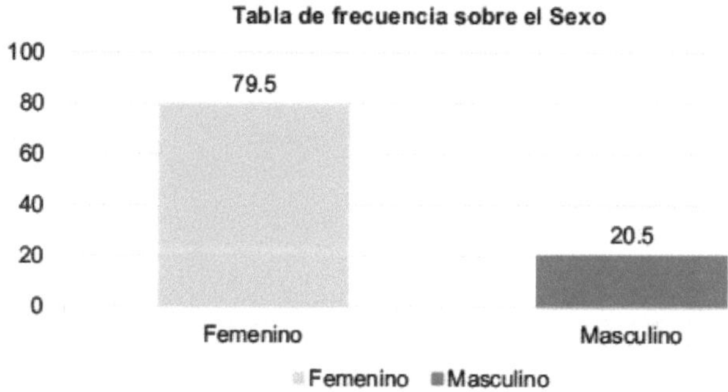

Source: SPSS Vs26

Interpretation and analysis: Table 2 and figure 2 show the distribution of the population according to sex; the trend indicates that 100 people (79.5%) are women and 27 people (20.5%) are men who presented with Trigeminal Neuralgia, consistent with the data on the Peruvian population according to sex from INEI in 2020, indicating a ratio of 99 males for every 100 females.

iii. Year of patient's admission to EsSalud-Cusco

***Table 11** Frequency table on the patient's year of admission to EsSalud - Cusco*

	Frequency	Percentage	Valid percentage	Cumulative percentage
2019	8	6,3	6,3	6,3
2020	56	44,1	44,1	50,4
Valid2021	45	35,4	35,4	85,8
2022	18	14,2	14,2	100,0
Total	127	100,0	100,0	

***Figure** 7 Patient's year of admission to EsSalud-Cusco*

Frequency table on the patient's Year of admission to EsSalud-Cusco

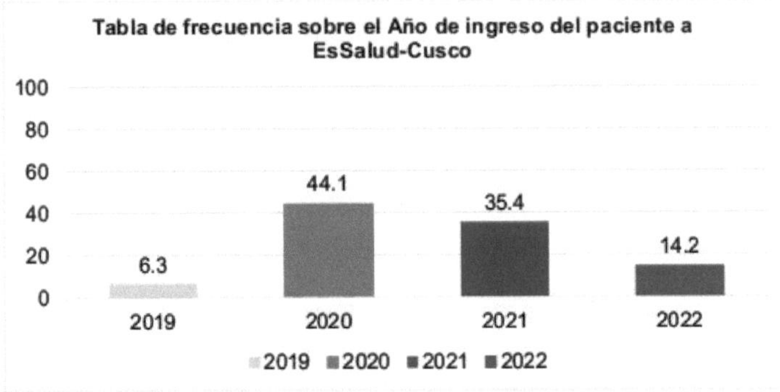

Source: SPSS Vs26

Interpretation and analysis: Table 3, Figure 3 shows the distribution of the population according to the year of admission of the patient to EsSalud-Cusco; the greatest trend is observed in 2020, where 56 people, representing 44.1% of the cases, presented with Trigeminal Neuralgia; in 2019, only 8 people, representing 6.3% of the cases; in 2021, 45 people, representing 35.4% of the cases; and in 2022, 18 people, representing 14.2% of the cases, presented with Trigeminal Neuralgia.3% of the cases, in the year 2021, 45 people, representing 35.4% of the cases and for the year 2022, 18 people, representing 14.2% of the patients, presented Trigeminal Neuralgia; predictably due to the fear of COVID-19.

- Dimension Etiological Factors

1. **Aetiological factors "COVID-19".**

a. **Positive test**

Table 12 *Frequency table on Aetiological factors of CO VID according to Positive Test*

	Frequency	Percentage	Valid percentage	Cumulative percentage
No Register	120	94,5	94,5	94,5
ValidIf	4	3,1	3,1	97,6
No	3	2,4	2,4	100,0
Total	127		100,0100,0	

Figure 8 *COVID Test Positive*

Frequency Table on Covid Aetiological Factors by Positive Test

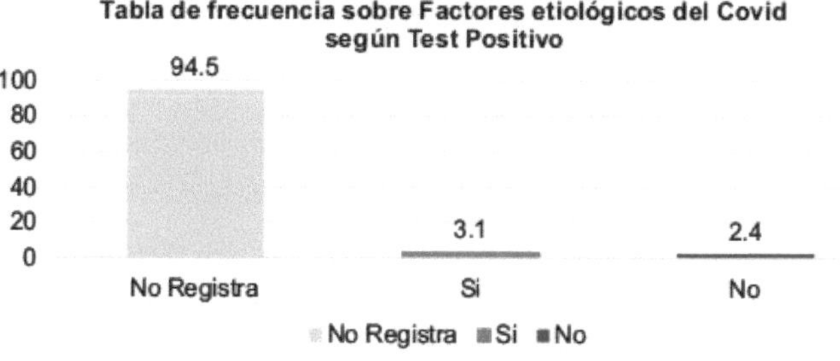

Source: SPSS Vs26

Interpretation and analysis: Table 4 Figure 4 shows the distribution of the population according to COVID-19 in relation to the Positive Test; the main trend is that 94.5% of the cases are not recorded in the computerised data.

In the hospital clinics, 3.1% did show a positive test and 2.4% of the cases did not establish a positive COVID-19 diagnosis.

b. Negative test

Table 13 *Frequency table on Aetiological factors of CO VID according to Negative Test*

		Frequency	Percentage	Valid percentage	Cumulative percentage
Valid	No Registra	121	95,3	95,3	95,3
	Yes	2	1,6	1,6	96,9
	No	4	3,1	3,1	100,0
	Total	127	100,0	100,0	

Figura 9 *COVID Test Negative*

Frequency table on Covid etiological factors according to Negative Test

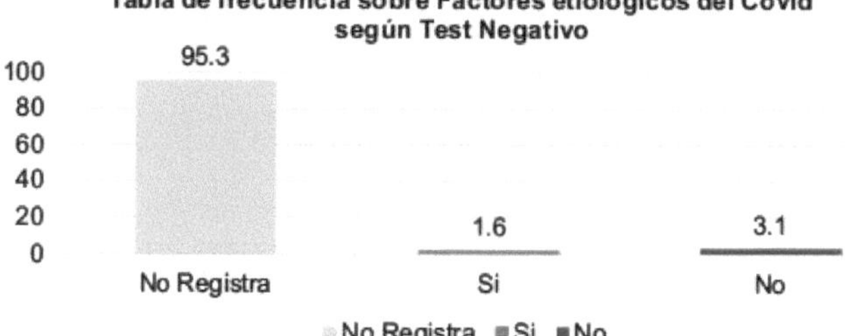

Source: SPSS Vs26

Interpretation and analysis: Table 5 Figure 5 shows the distribution of the population according to the COVID in relation to the Negative Test; the highest tendency is observed in 95.3% of the cases, in which no record is found, the highest tendency is observed in 95.3% of the cases, and the lowest tendency is observed in 95.3% of the cases, in which no record is found.

1.6% did show a negative test and 3.1% of the cases did not determine to have a negative test for COVID-19 diagnosis.

c.Vaccinated

Table 14 *Frequency table on Aetiological factors of CO VID according to whether Vaccinated*

	Frequency		Percentage	Valid percentage	Cumulative percentage
Valid	No Registra	125	98,4	98,4	98,4
	Yes		21,6	1,6	100,0
	Total	127	100,0	100,0	

Figura 10 *COVID Vaccinated*

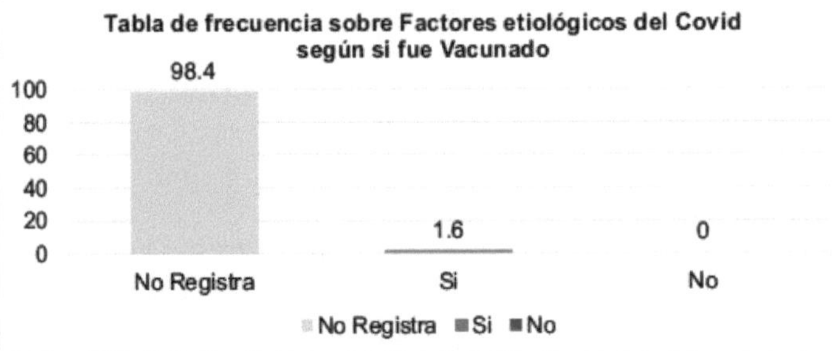

Source: SPSS Vs26

Interpretation and analysis: Table 6 Figure 6 shows the distribution of the population according to the COVID in relation to whether they received the vaccine; the main trend is that 98.4% of the cases are not registered, 1.6% do show vaccination in relation to the COVID-19 diagnosis; of these, a 51 year old patient of indigenous ethnicity, vaccinated with the 4ª dose, stated that she was diagnosed with secondary post-vaccination type TN.

d.Not vaccinated

Table 15 *Frequency Table on Aetiological Factors of CO VID Unvaccinated*

	Frequency		Percentage	Valid percentage	Cumulative percentage
Valid	No Registra	125	98,4	98,4	98,4
	No		21,6	1,6	100,0
	Total	127	100,0	100,0	

Figura 11 *COVID Not Vaccinated*

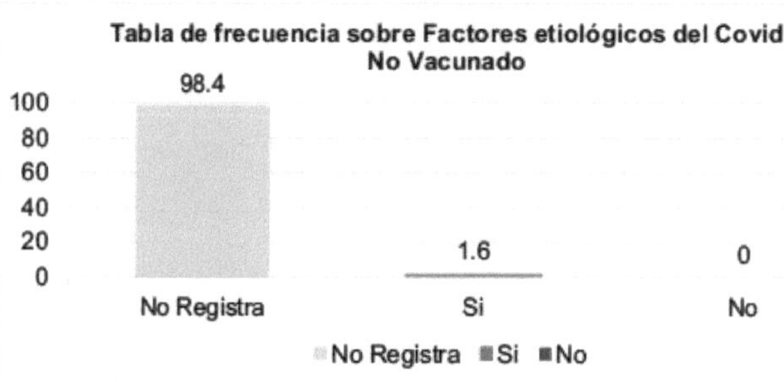

Source: SPSS Vs26

Interpretation and analysis: Table 6 Figure 6 shows the distribution of the population according to COVID in relation to the aetiological factors of COVID in unvaccinated persons; the main trend is that 98.4% of the cases are not registered, 1.6% show that they are unvaccinated in relation to the COVID-19 diagnosis.

i. Aetiological factors "Genetics or family ethnicity".

Table 16 *Frequency table on genetic-ethnic family history*

	Frequency	Percentage	Valid percentage	Cumulative percentage
White Ethnicity	0	0	0	0
Afro-descendant ethnicity	0	0	0	0
Mestizo Ethnicity	93	73,2	73,2	73,2
Valid Indigenous Ethnicity	34	26,8	26,8	100,0
Total	127	100,0	100,0	

Figure 12 *Genetic or ethnic family history*

Frequency of ethnic family backgrounds

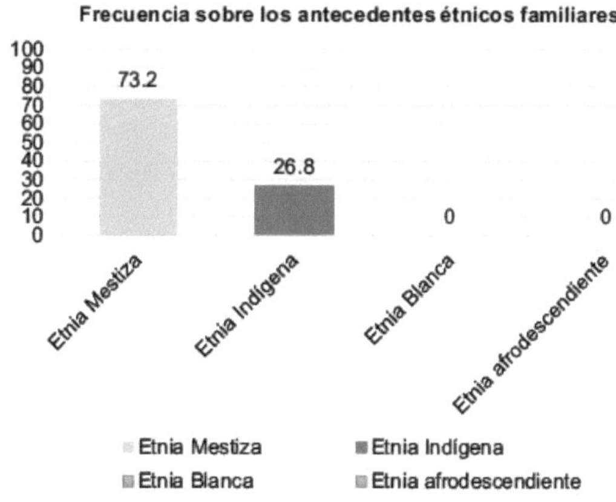

□ Ethnicity of African descent

Source: SPSS Vs26

Interpretation and analysis: Table 8, figure 8 shows the distribution of family genetic-ethnic antecedents; of the 100% of the cases studied, the greatest tendency is observed in 93 people, 73.2% of the cases studied, who are of mestizo ethnicity, while 34 people, representing 26.8%, are of indigenous ethnicity.

ii. **Aetiological factors "Tumour Cause".**

Table 17 *Frequency table for aetiological factors if they present Cause Tumour*

	Frequency		Percentage	Valid percentage	Cumulative percentage
Valid	No Registra	102	80,3	80,3	80,3
	Yes	10	7,9	7,9	88,2
	No	15	11,8	11,8	100,0
	Total	127	100,0	100,0	

Figure 13 *Tumour Cause*

Frequency table on etiological factors if present Tumour Cause

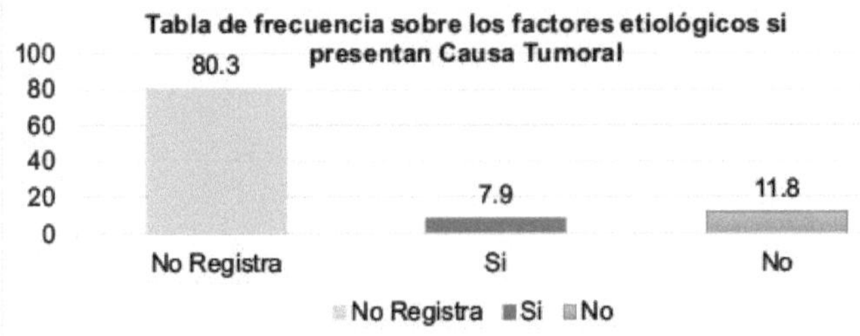

Source: SPSS Vs26

Interpretation and analysis: Table 8, figure 8 shows the distribution of the aetiological factors if they have a tumoural cause; of the 100% of the cases studied, the greatest tendency is observed in 102 people, comprising 80.3% of the cases studied, there are no tumoural cases, and 10 people, representing 7.9%, do have tumours and 15 people, representing 11.8%, do not have tumours.9% do present a tumour case and 15 people representing 11.8% do not present a tumour case; this casuistry as a genesis of trigeminal neuralgia, with surgical treatment and diagnosed by means of nuclear magnetic resonance NMR.

iii. **Aetiological factors "demyelination".**

Table 18 *Frequency table on aetiological factors Demyelination*

	Frequency	Percentage	Valid percentage	Cumulative percentage
No registers	114	89,8	89,8	89,8
ValidIf	6	4,7	4,7	94,5
No	7	5,5	5,5	100,0
Total	127	100,0	100,0	

Source: SPSS Vs26

Figure 14 *Demyelination*

Frequency table of aetiological factors
Demyelination

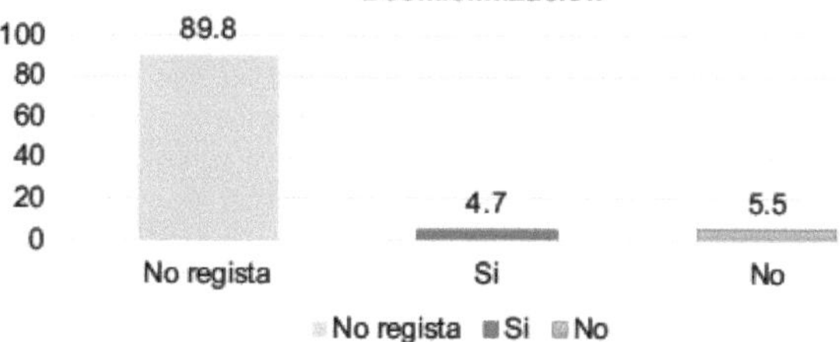

Source: SPSS Vs26

Interpretation and analysis: Table 9 Figure 9 shows the distribution of etiological factors in relation to demyelination; of the 100% of the cases studied, there is a greater tendency in 114 people representing 89.8% of the cases studied, who do not register etiological factors of demyelination in their clinical records, also 7 people representing 5.5% do not present demyelination and 6 people representing 4.7% do present demyelination. The 6 patients with a definitive diagnosis of demyelination are included in the 18 reports in which use was made of Magnetic Resonance Imaging (MRI); this apparatus had technical problems and has not been able to operate since 2020, as reported in the Adolfo Guevara Velasco Hospital.

iv. **Aetiological factors "Etiology unknown".**

Table 19 *Frequency table on aetiological factors "Etiology unknown".*

		Frequency	Percentage	Valid percentage	Cumulative percentage
Valid	No Registra	33	26,0	26,0	26,0
	Yes	70	55,1	55,1	81,1
	No	24	18,9	18,9	100,0
	Total	127	100,0	100,0	

Source: SPSS Vs26

Figure 15 Unknown aetiology

Frequency of aetiological factors "Etiology unknown unknown".

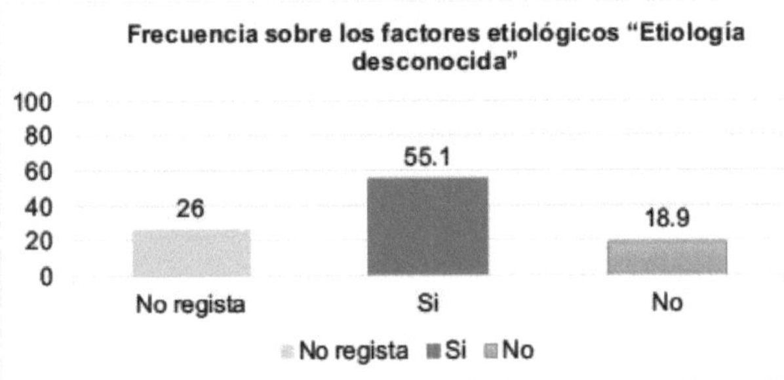

Interpretation and analysis: Table 14, figure 11 shows the distribution of aetiological factors in relation to "unknown aetiology"; of the 100% of the cases studied, there is a greater tendency for 70 people, representing 55.1% of the cases studied, to have an unknown aetiology, as well as 33 people, representing 26%, who do not have information of unknown aetiology and 24 people, representing 18.9%, who do not have an unknown aetiology.

4.1.1.2 Results for the Trigeminal Neuralgia Variable

- Etiology of Trigeminal Neuralgia

i. Type of Trigeminal Neuralgia

Table 20 *Frequency table on Type of Trigeminal Neurology*

	Frequency	Percentage	Valid percentage	Cumulative percentage
Classical	40	31,5	31,5	31,5
Secondary	13	10,2	10,2	41,7
Valid				
Idiopathic	44	34,6	34,6	76,4
No Registra	30	23,6	23,6	100,0
Total	127	100,0	100,0	

Figure 16 *Type of Trigeminal Neuralgia*

Frequency table on the Type of Trigeminal Neuralgia

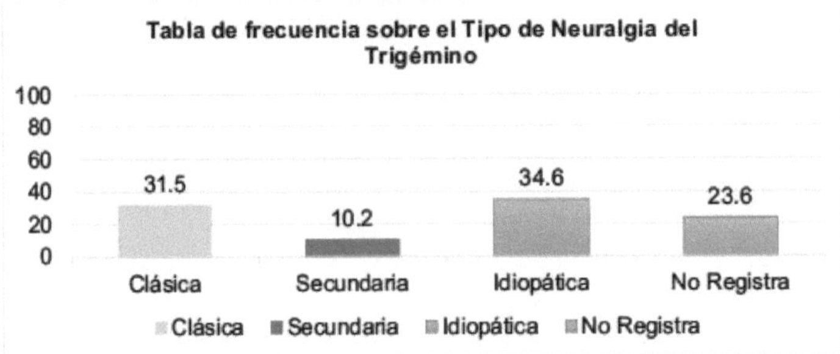

Interpretation and analysis: Table 11 Figure 11 shows the distribution of the Type of

Trigeminal Neuralgia; of the 100% of the cases studied, the highest tendency is observed in 44 people, 34.6% of the cases studied.In the same way, 40 people, representing 31.5% of the cases studied, recorded as idiopathic; 13 people recorded a type of trigeminal neuralgia secondary to 10.2% and 30 people did not record any information in 23.6% of the cases.

- Pain Scales

i. Visual Analogue Scale (VAS)

Table 21 *Frequency table on the visual analogue scale (VAS)*

		Frequency	Percentage	Valid percentage	Cumulative percentage
Valid os	Pain Soft 1-3		75,5	5,5	5,5
	Pain moderate 4-6	13	10,2	10,2	15,7
	Pain intense 7-10	75	59,1	59,1	74,8
	No Register 0	32	25,2	25,2	100,0
	Total		127100,0	100,0	

Figure 17 *Visual Analogue Scale (VAS)*

Frequency table on the Visual Analogue Scale (VAS)

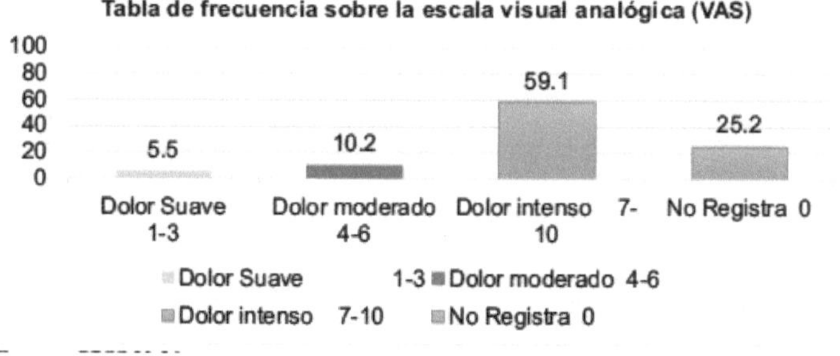

Source: SPSS Vs26

Interpretation and analysis: Table 12, figure 12 shows the distribution on the visual analogue scale (VAS) of 100% of the cases studied. The main trend is that 75 people (59.1% of the cases studied) have severe pain, 13 people (10.2%) have moderate pain, 7 people (5.5%) have mild pain and 32 people (25.2%) have no information in their clinical data.

i. Scale for mentally handicapped and other criteria a. Grimacing

Table 22 *Frequency table on the scale for mentally handicapped and other criteria Grimaces*

Frequency	Percentage	Valid percentage	Cumulative percentage

	No Registra	122	96,1	96,1	96,1
Valid	No		53,9	3,9	100,0
	Total	127	100,0	100,0	

Figure 18 Grimaces

Frequency table on the mentally handicapped scale and other criteria Grimaces

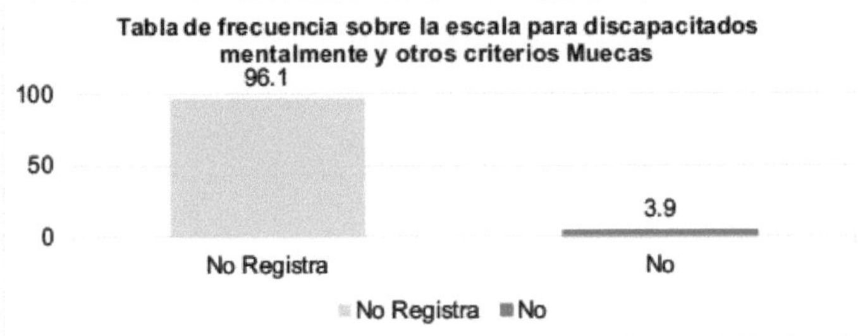

Source: SPSS Vs26

Interpretation and analysis: Table 13, figure 13 shows the distribution on the scale for the mentally handicapped on the criterion Grimacing; 96.1% of the cases studied do not record information and there are 5 people, representing 3.9%, who indicate that they grimaced in the face of intense pain.

b. Pupillary Dilatation

Table 23 *Frequency table on the scale for the mentally handicapped on the criterion Pupillary dilatation*

	Frequency		Percentage	Valid percentage	Cumulative percentage
Valid	No Register	122	96,1	96,1	96,1
	No	5	3,9	3,9	100,0
	Total	127	100,0	100,0	

Figure 19 *Pupillary dilation*

Frequency table on the scale for the mentally handicapped on the pupillary dilation criterion

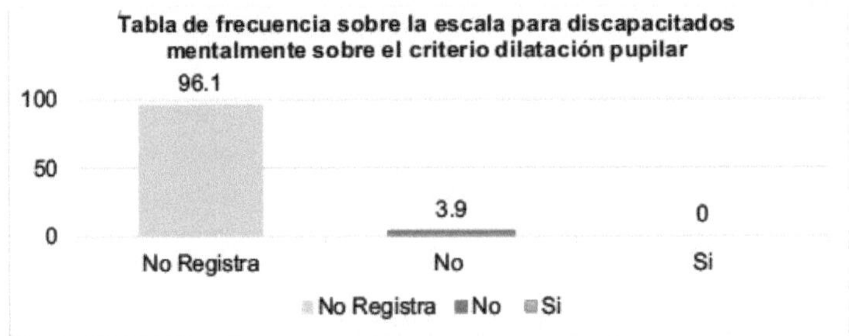

Source: SPSS Vs26

Interpretation and analysis: Table 19, figure 16 shows the distribution on the scale for the mentally handicapped according to the criterion pupillary dilatation 96.1% of the studied cases do not register information and 5 persons comprising 3.9 % of the studied cases indicate that they do not present pupillary dilatation. Perhaps, they did not notice the eye language in cases of severe pain.

c. Frequency of pain

Table 24 *Frequency table on the scale for mentally handicapped and other criteria Frequency of pain*

		Frequency	Percentage	Valid percentage	Cumulative percentage
Valid	No Registra	80	63,0	63,0	63,0
	Daily	38	29,9	29,9	92,9
	Weekly		97,1	7,1	100,0
	Total	127	100,0	100,0	

Figure 20 *Frequency of pain*

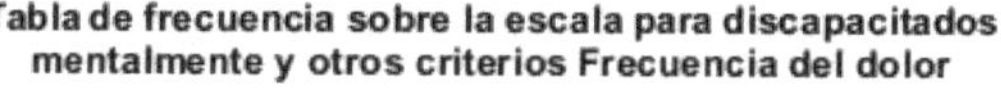

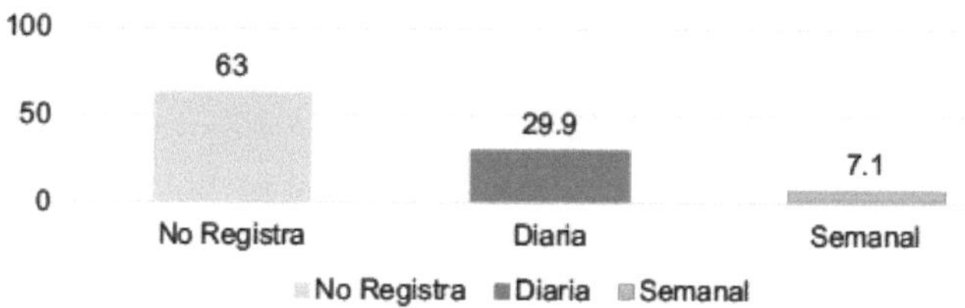

Fuente: SPSS Vs26

Interpretation and analysis: Table 14, figure 14 shows the distribution on the scale for the mentally handicapped, according to the criterion Frequency of pain, 63% of the cases studied do not record any information, 38 people, or 29.9% of the cases studied, indicate that they have pain on a daily basis, and 9 people, or 7.1%, indicate that the pain occurs on a weekly basis.

d. Referrals to Limes

Table 25 *Frequency table on the scale for mentally handicapped and Referred to Lima*

		Frequency	Percentage	Valid percentage	Cumulative percentage
Valid	No Registra	28	22,0	22,0	22,0
	No	99	78,0	78,0	100,0
	Total	127	100,0	100,0	

Frequency table on the mentally disabled scale and were referred to Lima.

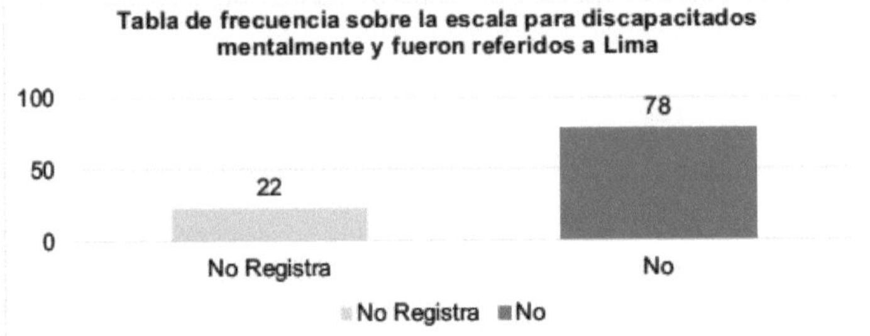

Source: SPSS Vs26

Interpretation and analysis: Table 15, figure 15 shows the distribution on the scale for the mentally handicapped; 38 people (78% of the cases studied) indicated that they were not referred to Lima, and 22 people (22%) did not register any information.

ii. **Alcantara and Gonzalez pain test a. Affected branches**

Table 26 *Frequency table on the pain scale according to affected Branches*

	Frequency	Percentage	Valid percentage	Cumulative percentage	
No Register	67	52,8	52,8	52,8	
V1		3	2,4	2,455,1	
ValidV2	19	15,0	15,0	70,1	
V3	14	11,0	11,0	81,1	
V1/V2/V3	24	18,9	18,9		100,0
Total	127		100,0	100,0	

Figure 22 *Affected branches*

Frequency table on the pain scale according to affected branches

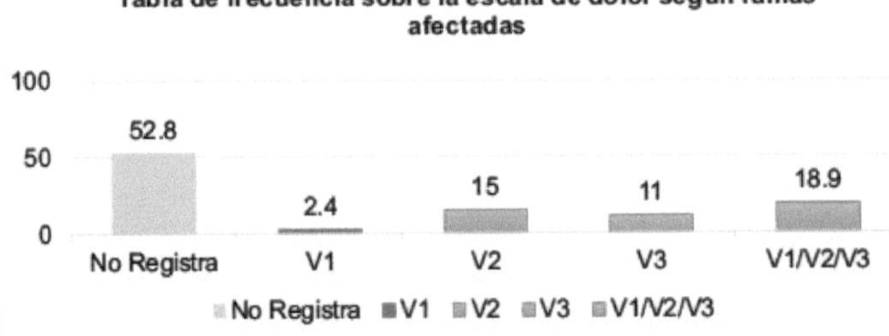

Source: SPSS Vs26

Interpretation and analysis: Table 16, figure 16 shows the distribution of the pain scale according to the branches affected, where 67 patients, representing 52.8 % of the cases studied, did not record any information, 24 people, comprising 18.9 % of the cases studied indicated that they presented pain in branches V1, V2 and V3, likewise 15 people, representing 15%, indicated that the pain was present in V2, 14 people, representing 11%, indicated that the pain manifested itself in V3 and finally 3 people, representing 2.4%, indicated that the pain was triggered in V1; most probably due to psychological factors such as stress and anxiety developed during the COVID-19 pandemic.

b. Facial side affected by pain

***Table 27** Frequency table on the pain scale by affected side*

	Frequency	Percentage	Valid percentage	Cumulative percentage
No Registra	31	24,4	24,4	24,4
Right	41	32,3	32,3	56,7
Left	45	35,4	35,4	92,1
Valid				
Both sides	10	7,9	7,9	100,0
Total	127	100,0	100,0	

***Figure 23** Facial side affected*

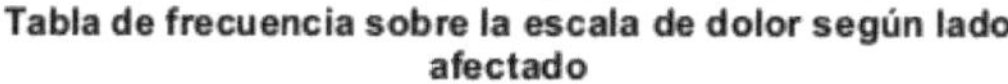

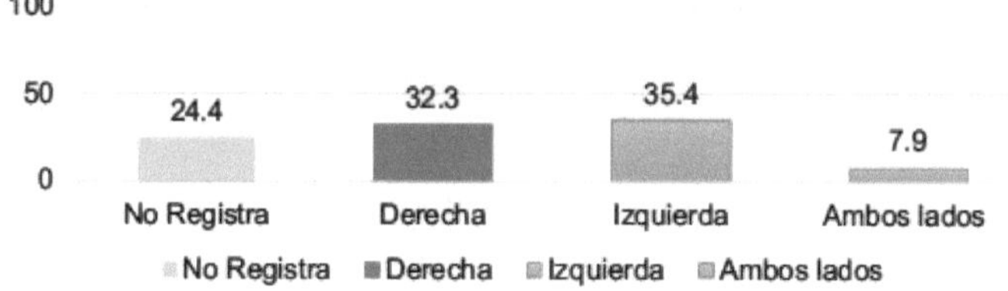

Interpretation and analysis: Table 17 and figure 17 show the distribution of the pain scale according to the affected side, where 24.4% of the cases studied did not register any information, 41 people, which represents 32.3% of the cases studied, indicated that the pain was on the right side, 45 people, which represents 35.4%, indicated that the pain developed on the left side and 10 people, which represents 7.9%, indicated that the pain was on both sides.

c. Onset of pain

***Table 28** Frequency table on the pain scale according to Start of pain*

	Frequency	Percentage	Valid percentage	Cumulative percentage
Soft	11	8,7	8,7	8,7
Moderate		97,1	7,1	15,7
ValidosBrusco	71	55,9	55,9	71,7
No Registra	36	28,3	28,3	100,0
Total		127100,0	100,0	

Figure 24 *Onset of pain*

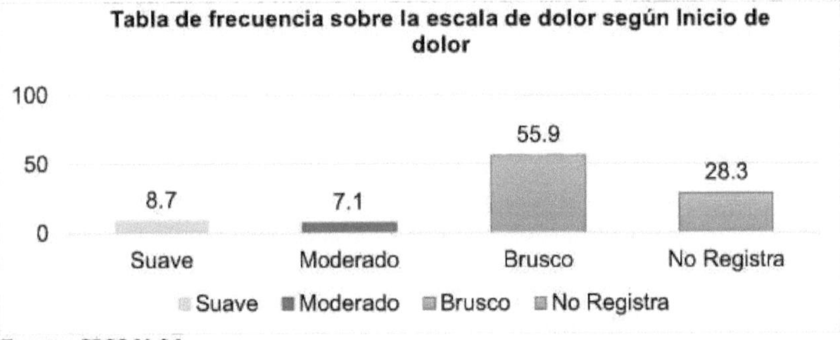

Fuente: SPSS Vs26

Interpretation and analysis: Table 18 and figure 18 show the distribution of how the pain scale starts; 55.9% of the cases studied indicate that it starts abruptly, 28.3% of the cases studied do not record any information, likewise 11 people (8.7%) indicate that the pain was of mild onset and 9 people (7.1%) indicate that the pain is moderate.

d. **Duration**

Table 29 *Frequency table on the pain scale according to Duration*

		Frequency	Percentage	Valid percentage	Cumulative percentage
	Sec. to 2 min.	14	11,0	11,0	11.0
-\ 1i rlrtc;	More than 2 minutes	13	10,2	10,2	21,3
os	No Registra	100	78,7	78,7	100,0
	Total	127	100,0	100,0	

Figure 25 *Duration*

Frequency table on the pain scale according to duration

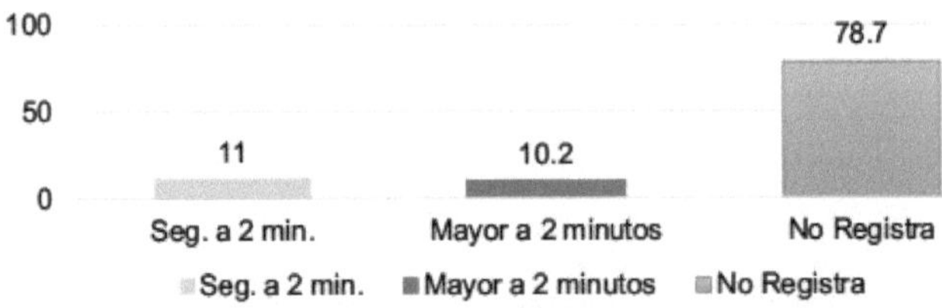

Source: SPSS Vs26

Interpretation and analysis: Table 19 and figure 19 show the distribution of the pain scale according to duration, where it can be seen that in 100 people (78.7%) there is no record of the duration, 11% of the cases studied indicate that the pain lasts less than 2 minutes, and 13 people (10.2%) indicate that the pain lasts more than 2 minutes.

e. **Type of pain**

Table 30 *Frequency table on Type of pain*

	Frequency	Percentage	Valid percentage	Cumulative percentage

Provoked	35	27,6	27,6	27,6
Spontaneous Valid	63	49,6	49,6	77,2
No Registra	29	22,8	22,8	100,0
Total	127	100,0	100,0	

Figure 26 *Type of pain*

Frequency table on type of pain

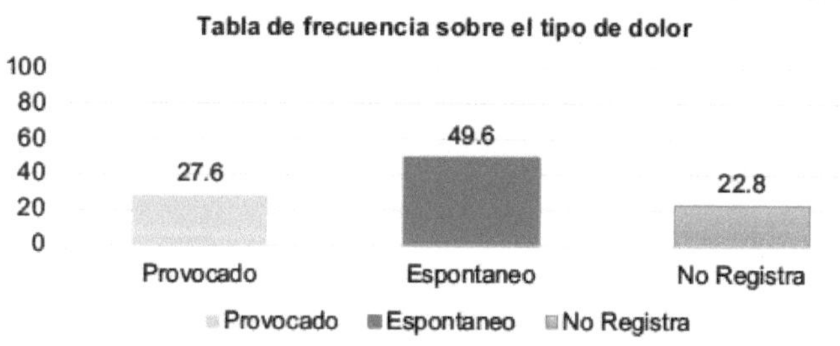

Source: SPSS Vs26

Interpretation and analysis: Table 20 and figure 20 show the distribution of the type of pain, where it can be seen that in 69 people (49.6%) the pain was spontaneous, 35 people (27.6% of the cases studied) indicated that the pain was provoked, and 29 cases (22.8%) did not register any information.

f. **Stimulus triggered**

Table 31 *Frequency table on elicited stimuli*

	Frequency	Percentage	Valid percentage	Cumulative percentage
Safe mechanic	71	55,9	55,9	55,9
Movements				
Valid	20	15,7	15,7	71,7
No Registra	36	28,3	28,3	100,0
Total	127	100,0	100,0	

Figure 27 *Triggered stimulus*

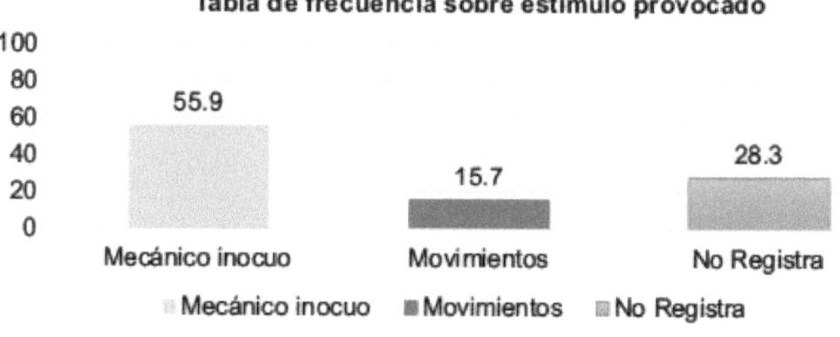

Fuente: SPSS Vs26

Interpretation and analysis: Table 21 and figure 21 show the distribution of the frequency of the provoked stimulus; where it is observed that 71 people, representing 55.9%, the frequency of pain is mechanical and innocuous, 20 people, equivalent to 15.7% of the cases studied, indicate that the frequency is in movements, and 36 of the cases, representing 28.3%, do not record any information in their clinical data.

g. Pain between paroxysms

Table 32 *Frequency Table on Pain between paroxysms*

		Frequency	Percentage	Valid percentage	Cumulative percentage
Valid	No Registra	69	54,3	54,3	54,3
	Yes	48	37,8	37,8	92,1
	No	10	7,9	7,9	100,0
	Total		127100,0	100,0	

Figure 28 *Pain between paroxysms*

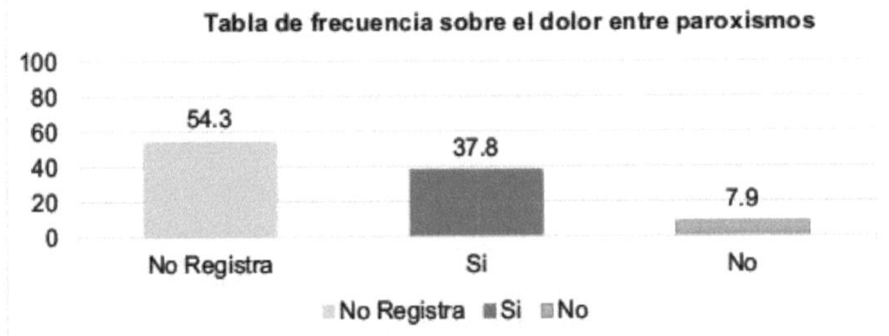

Fuente: SPSS Vs26

Interpretation and analysis: Table 22 and figure 22 show the distribution of the frequency of pain between paroxysms; where it is observed that 69 of the cases, which represents 54.3%, do not register information, 48 people, equivalent to 37.8% of the cases studied, indicate that there is pain between paroxysms and finally 10 people, equivalent to 7.9% of the cases studied, indicate that there is no pain between paroxysms.

h. Additional continuous pain

Table 33 *Frequency table on Additional continuous pain*

		Frequency	Percentage	Valid percentage	Cumulative percentage
Valid	No Registra	48	37,8	37,8	37,8
	Yes	70	55,1	55,1	92,9
	No		97,1	7,1	100,0
	Total	127	100,0	100,0	

Figure 29 *Additional continuous pain*

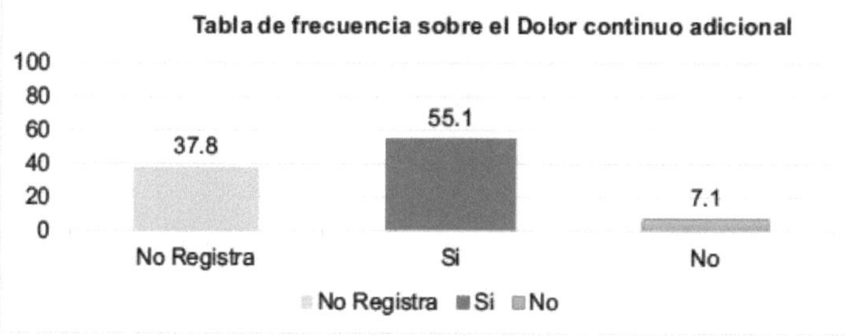

Interpretation and analysis: Table 23 and figure 23 show the distribution of the frequency of additional continuous pain; where it can be seen that 48 of the cases, representing 37.8%, do not record information, 70 people, equivalent to 55.1% of the cases studied, indicate that there is additional continuous pain and finally 10 people, equivalent to 7.1% of the cases studied, indicate that there is no additional continuous pain.

4.2 Hypothesis testing

4.2.1 General hypothesis

a. Null hypothesis (Ho). There is no common etiology of trigeminal neuralgia in patients seen in EsSalud Cusco from January 2019 to August 2022.

b. Alternating hypothesis (H1). There is a more common etiology of trigeminal neuralgia in patients seen in EsSalud Cusco from January 2019 to August 2022.

c. Level of significance (a):

$$\alpha = 5\%,\ X^2_t = X\ 2\text{crítico} = 3{,}6871$$

d. Statistical Test:

$$X2\ c = X\ 2\ calc = \Sigma(oi - ei)^2 / ei,\ X2\ c = 1{,}195a$$

Where:

- oi = Observed value
- ei = Expected value
- X2c = Value of the statistic calculated with data from the surveys and processed using SPSS Vs28 statistical software, and should be compared with the values associated with the significance level indicated in the contingency table N° 24.

a. Decision: Ho is rejected.

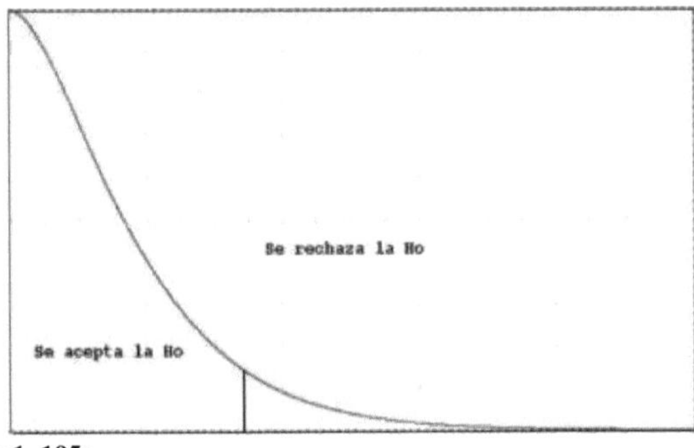

X^2 t = 3.6871 X^2 c= 1, 195a

Interpretation:

With a significance level of 5%, the null hypothesis is rejected and the alternate hypothesis is accepted, concluding that "There is an average relationship in the most common aetiology of trigeminal neuralgia in patients treated in EsSalud Cusco from January 2019 to August 2022", for which the calculations are attached, consisting of the contingency table No. 24 and the result of the Chi-square statistical test.

Chi-Square Test

***Table 34** Contingency table on the most common aetiology of trigeminal neuralgia in patients seen in ESSALUD Cusco from January 2019 to August 2022.*

		V2 TRIGEMINAL NEURALGIA			Total
		Low ratio	Average ratio	High ratio	
V1 MOST COMMON AETIOLOGY	Low ratio	0	42	7	49
	Average ratio	1	68	8	77
	High ratio	0	1	0	1
Total		1	111	15	127

***Table 35** Chi-square tests*

	Value	gl	Sig. asymptotic (bilateral)
Pearson's Chi-square	1,195[a]	4	,879
Likelihood ratio	1,653	4	,799
Linear by linear association	,799	1	,371
N of valid cases	127		

a. 5 cells (55.6%) have an expected frequency of less than 5. The minimum expected frequency is ,01.

4.2.2 Specific hypotheses

Specific Hypothesis 1

a. Null hypothesis (Ho). There is no relationship between TN and age in patients seen in EsSalud Cusco from January 2019 to August 2022.

b. Alternating hypothesis (H1). There is a relationship between TN and age in patients seen in EsSalud Cusco from January 2019 to August 2022.

c. Level of significance (a):

$$\alpha = 5\%,\ X2t = X2critical = 5{,}3481$$

d. Statistical Test:

$X2\ c = X\ 2\ calc = \Sigma(oi - ei)^2 / ei, X2\ c = 10{,}587a$

Where:

- oi = Observed value
- ei = Expected value
- X2c = Value of the statistic calculated with data from the surveys and processed using SPSS Vs28 statistical software, and should be compared with the values associated with the significance level indicated in the contingency table N° 26.

b. Decision: Ho is rejected.

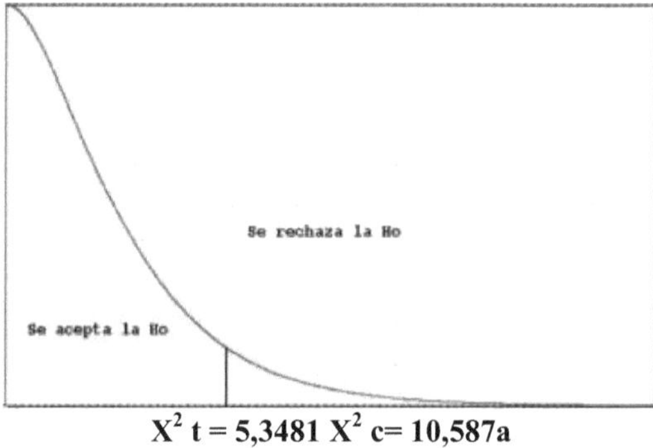

$X^2\ t = 5{,}3481\ X^2\ c = 10{,}587a$

Interpretation:

With a significance level of 5%, the null hypothesis is rejected and the alternate hypothesis is accepted, concluding that "There is a relationship between TN and age in patients seen in EsSalud Cusco from January 2019 to August 2022", for which the calculations are attached, consisting of the contingency table No. 26 and the result of the Chi-square statistical test.

- Chi-Square Test

Table 36 *Contingency table on whether there is a relationship between TN and age in patients seen in EsSalud Cusco from January 2019 to August 2022.*

Predisposing Factors by Age

	20 a 40 years	41 a 60 years	61 to 80 years	81 to 95 years	Total
Low ratio	10	24	14	1	49

V1 Most Common Aetiology	Average ratio	6	28	39	4	77
	High ratio	0	1	0	0	1
Total		16	53	53	5	127

***Table 37** Chi-square tests*

	Value	gl	Sig. asymptotic (bilateral)
Pearson's Chi-square	10,587[a]	6	,102
Likelihood ratio	11,005	6	,088
Linear by linear association	7,643	1	,006
N of valid cases	127		

a. 6 cells (50.0%) have an expected frequency of less than 5. The minimum expected frequency is ,04.

Specific Hypothesis 2

a. Null hypothesis (Ho). There is no relationship between TN and gender in patients seen in EsSalud Cusco from January 2019 to August 2022.

b. Alternating hypothesis (H2). There is a relationship between TN and gender in patients seen in EsSalud Cusco from January 2019 to August 2022.

c. Level of significance (a):

$$\alpha = 5\%, X^2\ t = X2\text{critical} = 1.3863$$

d. Statistical test:

$$X2\ c = X\ 2\ calc = \Sigma(oi - ei)^2 / ei, X2\ c = 20{,}847a$$

Where:

- oi = Observed value
- ei = Expected value
- X2c = Value of the statistic calculated with data from the surveys and processed using SPSS Vs28 statistical software, and should be compared with the values associated with the significance level indicated in the contingency table N° 28.

c. Decision: Ho is rejected.

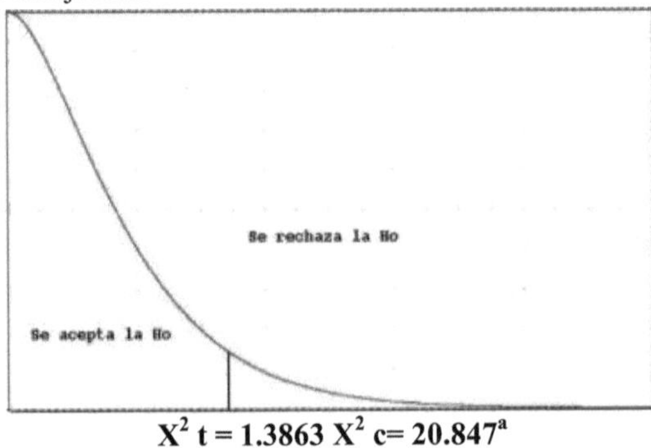

X^2 t = 1.3863 X^2 c= 20.847[a]

Interpretation:

With a significance level of 5%, the null hypothesis is rejected and the alternative hypothesis is accepted, concluding that "There is a relationship between TL and gender in patients attended in EsSalud Cusco from January 2019 to August 2022", for which the calculations are attached, consisting of the contingency table No. 28 and the result of the Chi-square statistical test.

- Chi-Square Test

Table 38 *Contingency table on the relation between TN and gender in patients seen in EsSalud Cusco from January 2019 to August 2022.*

		Gender of patients seen		Total
		Female	Male	
V1 ETIOLOGY MORE COMMON	Low ratio		48	048
	Average ratio		51	2677
	High ratio		1	01
Total			100	26126

Table 39 *Chi-square tests*

	Value	gl	Sig. asymptotic (bilateral)
Pearson's Chi-square	20,847[a]	2	,000
Likelihood ratio	29,809	2	,000
Linear by linear association	18,107	1	,000
N of valid cases	126		

a. 2 cells (33.3%) have an expected frequency of less than 5. The minimum expected frequency is ,21.

Specific Hypothesis 3

a. Null hypothesis (Ho). There is no relationship between TN and COVID in patients seen in EsSalud Cusco from January 2019 to August 2022.

b. Alternating hypothesis (H3). There is a relationship between TN and COVID in patients treated at EsSalud Cusco from January 2019 to August 2022.

c. Level of significance (a):

α= : 5%, X^2 t = *X* 2crftico =3,**3660**

d. Statistical test:

X2 c = *X* 2 *calc* = Σ(oi – ei $)^2$ / ei, X2 c = 66,015[a]

Where:

- oi = Observed value
- ei = Expected value
- X2c = Value of the statistic calculated with data from the surveys and processed using SPSS Vs28 statistical software, and should be compared with the values associated with the significance level indicated in the contingency table N° 32.

d. Decision: Ho is rejected.

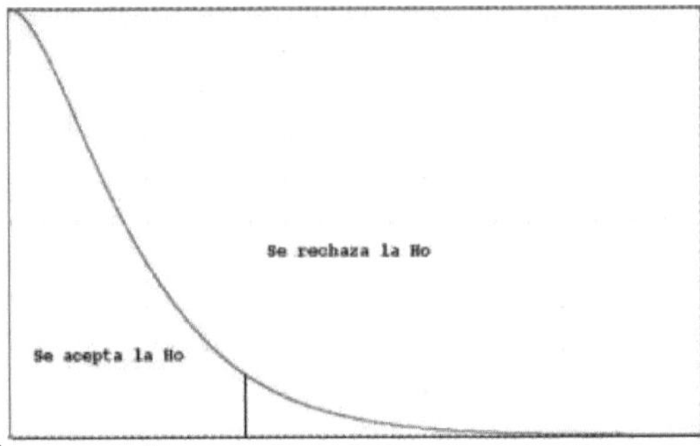

X^2 t = 3.3660 X^2 c= 66.015[a]

Interpretation:
With a significance level of 5%, the null hypothesis is rejected and the alternative hypothesis is accepted, concluding that "There is a relationship between TN and COVID in patients treated in EsSalud Cusco from January 2019 to August 2022", for which the calculations are attached, consisting of the contingency table No. 32 and the result of the Chi-square statistical test.

- Chi-Square Test

Table 40 *Contingency table on the relationship between TN and CO VID in patients seen in EsSalud Cusco from January 2019 to August 2022.*

		COVID			
		Relation low	Relation half	Relation high	Total
V1_ETIOLOGLA.	_mAS_COMUNRelacion490049 low				
	Average ratio	72	4	177	
	High ratio	0	0	11	
Total		121	4	2127	

Table 41 *Chi-square tests*

	Value	gl	Sig. asymptotic (bilateral)
Pearson's Chi-square	66,015[a]	4	,000
Likelihood ratio	13,964	4	,007
Linear by linear association	8,682	1	,003
N of valid cases127			

a. 7 cells (77.8%) have an expected frequency of less than 5. The minimum expected frequency is ,02.

Specific Hypothesis 4

a. Null hypothesis (Ho). There is no relationship between TN and genetics in patients seen in EsSalud Cusco from January 2019 to August 2022.

b. Alternating hypothesis (H4). There is a relationship between TN and genetics in patients treated in EsSalud Cusco from January 2019 to August 2022.

c. Level of significance (a):

$\alpha =$: 5%, X^2 t = X2critical =5.9915

d. Statistical Test:

X2 c = X 2 *calc* = Σ(oi – ei)² / ei, X2 c = 4,124ª Where:

- oi = Observed value
- ei = Expected value
- X2c = Value of the statistic calculated with data from the surveys and processed with SPSS statistical software.

Vs28, and should be compared with the values associated with the significance level given in contingency table No. 32 e. Decision: Ho is rejected.

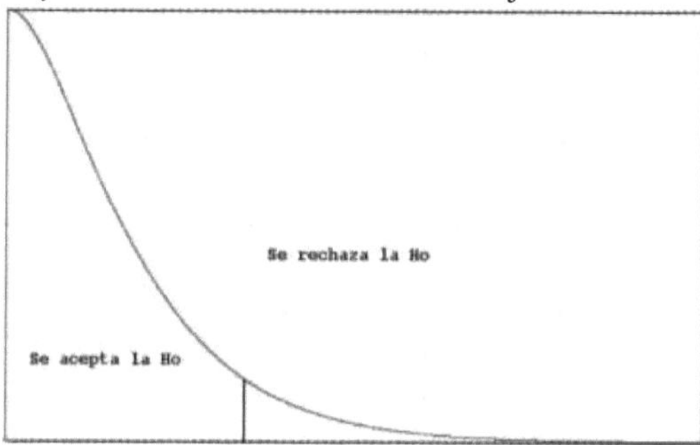

X^2 t = 1.3863 X^2 c= 4.124ª

Interpretation:

With a significance level of 5%, the null hypothesis is rejected and the alternative hypothesis is accepted, concluding that "There is a relationship between NT and genetics in patients treated in EsSalud Cusco from January 2019 to August 2022", for which the calculations are attached, consisting of the contingency table No. 32 and the result of the Chi-square statistical test.

Table 42 *Contingency table on the relationship between TN and CO VID in patients seen in EsSalud Cusco from January 2019 to August 2022.*

		Aetiological factors Genetics			
		Mestizo Ethnicity	Indigenous Ethnicity	Total	
V1 Most Common Aetiology	Low ratio	39	10	49	
	Average ratio	54	23	77	
	High ratio		0	1	1
Total		93		34	127

Table 43 *Chi-square tests*

		Value	gl	Sig. asymptotic (bilateral)
Pearson's Chi-square		4,124ª	2	,127
Likelihood ratio		4,076	2	,130
Linear by linear association		2,355	1	,125
N of valid cases	127			

a. 2 cells (33.3%) have an expected frequency of less than 5. The minimum expected frequency is ,27.

Specific Hypothesis 5

a. Null hypothesis (Ho). There is no relationship between TN and tumours in patients seen in EsSalud Cusco from January 2019 to August 2022.

b. Alternating hypothesis (H5). There is a relationship between TN and tumours in patients treated at EsSalud Cusco from January 2019 to August 2022.

c. Level of significance (a):

$$\alpha = 5\%, X^2 t = X 2crftico = \mathbf{9,4877}$$

d. Statistical test:

$$\mathbf{X2\ c = X\ 2\ calc = \Sigma(oi - ei)^2 / ei, X2\ c = 22,413^a}$$

Where:

- oi = Observed value
- ei = Expected value
- X2c = Value of the statistic calculated with data from the surveys and processed using SPSS Vs28 statistical software, and should be compared with the values associated with the significance level indicated in the contingency table N° 34.

f. Decision: Ho is rejected.

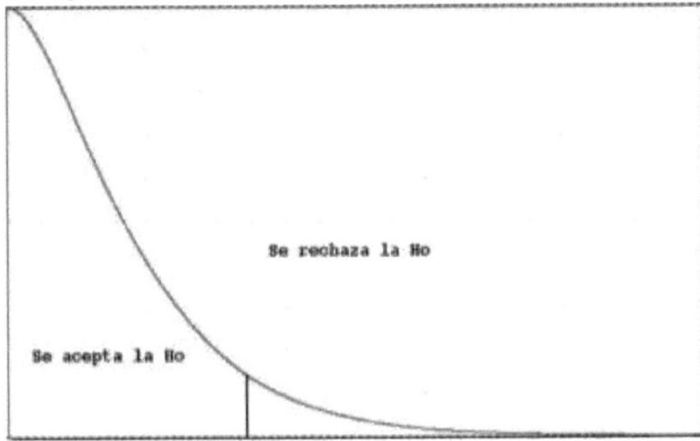

$\mathbf{X^2\ t = 3.3567\ X^2\ c = 22.413^a}$

Interpretation:

With a significance level of 5%, the null hypothesis is rejected and the alternative hypothesis is accepted, concluding that "There is a relationship between TN and tumours in patients treated in EsSalud Cusco from January 2019 to August 2022", for which the calculations are attached, consisting of the contingency table No. 34 and the result of the Chi-square statistical test.

***Table 44** Contingency table on the relationship between TN and tumours in patients seen in EsSalud Cusco from January 2019 to August 2022.*

	Tumour Cause			Total
	No Registra	Yes	No	
Low ratio V1 Aetiology More	48	0	149	
Average ratio Common	54	10	1377	

High ratio	00	1	1
Total	102 10	15	127

***Table 45** Chi-square tests*

	Value	gl	Sig. asymptotic (bilateral)
Pearson's Chi-square	22,413[a]		4,000
Likelihood ratio	24,477		4,000
Linear by linear association	15,748		1,000
N of valid cases	127		

a. 4 cells (44.4%) have an expected frequency of less than 5. The minimum expected frequency is ,08.

4.3. Presentation of the Discussion of the Results

Regarding the most common aetiology: For Boto (2010), it is rare for TN to present as trigeminal status or a rapid succession of tic-like spasms, provoked by any stimulus (5). Meanwhile Beltran and Freyre (2012), 86% of patients consulted a physician at the first attacks of pain. The specialists consulted before the diagnosis of TN were: primary care physicians (PCP) 43.1%, dentists 30.4%, otolaryngologists 3.9%, neurosurgeons 3.9%, neurologists or headache specialists 14.7%, others 8%. The final diagnosis was made by a neurologist or headache specialist 85.3%, and the mean interval between the onset of the disease and diagnosis by a specialist was 10.8 ± 21.2 months (1). According to Alcantara and Sanchez (2016), the incidence of TN is 413% (18). On the other hand, Inoyatova et al. (2021), established the following supposed aetiological factors for the development of the disease: frequent hypothermia 26% and concomitant diseases in patients with TN hypertonic disease 31% (25). To conclude, Smith et al (2021). There is no clear candidate genesis, (6).

According to the most common aetiology of Trigeminal Neuralgia (TN), considered in this scientific research study; as a predisposing factor, there was an average relationship, the most prominent being: female sex at 79.As a predisposing factor, there was an average relationship, the most prominent being: female sex at 79.5%, as indicated by a history of investigation; followed by age between 41 and 80 years at 41.7%; finally, the year 2020 at 41% and the lowest range was 2019 at 6.3%, most likely due to the anxiety and stress caused by the quarantine due to the COVID-19 pandemic. As an aetiological factor: the unknown aetiology was shown to be of the highest proportion at 55.1%, mainly due to the disuse of the medical device for nuclear magnetic resonance imaging (MRI); then the mestizo ethnic-genetic component at 73.2%; the tumour origin at 7.9%, diagnosed with MRI in 14.9% of the cases.9% diagnosed by MRI in 14 patients; demyelination in 6 patients, representing 4.7%; finally, COVID in 3.1 % of cases, including a 51 year old patient, who manifested trigeminal neuralgia after vaccination with the 4[a] anti COVID dose. As for the Peruvian ethnic group, it is a range of origins, with a female majority, 99 men for every 100 women, according to INEI data for 2020.

At the national level in terms of age: Vasquez (2020), TN is more common among people aged 60 to 69 years, and unilaterally on the right side in 59.5% of cases (14). Internationally, according to Boto (2010), it occurs over 50 years around 63 years, the V2 and V3 branches are the most injured at 42% of cases, the V2 branch alone at 20%, the V3 branch alone at 17% and V1 and V2 together at 14%, and V1, V2 and V3 at 5% and V1 alone at 2% (5).(5) According to Alcantara and Gonzales (2017), he relates the story of a 49-year-old patient with a 10-year history of acute, dull, constant pain from mechanical and sensory stimuli in the third branch of the trigeminal nerve (20). On the other hand, Grin et al. (2018), highlight the case of a 73-year-old patient, who underwent root canal treatment in 22, 23 and 25, the latter with apicoectomy, in addition to root canals in 24 and 26, when the real diagnosis was TN type I (13). Subsequently Ayele et al. (2020), the age group of the 61 participants ranged from 21 to 78 years; 68.9 % reported involvement of the right facial side, where the most common branch was the mandibular 47.5 %; (90.2 %) of the patients fulfilled criteria for classic TN and 9.8 % had symptomatic TN. Most participants reported mixed types of pain, such as burning, lancinating and electric shock-like (21). As for Jaramillo and Mendoza (2020), they identified 39 patients with TN, who reported according to age group: age 50-90 years, involvement of the facial sinus area in 72% or 28 cases; with severe unilateral pain in the maxillary branch or V2 on Valleix examination, with 47% or 28 patients (22). Thus Inoyatova et al. (2021), by age range, middle-aged and elderly patients suffer more often from TN at 66.7%; patients of different ages react heterogeneously to the pain syndrome. Therefore, the clinical picture of TN is determined by lesions in the branches, the most specific symptoms of which are the presence of trigger zones for the development of pain (25). From another perspective, Lara C. (2021), it develops in people over 50 years of age, while for its treatment, the drugs in order of choice are: Carbamazepine, lamotrigine, baclofen, gabapentin, pregabalin, botulinum toxin; finally, waiting for a better tolerated drug (26). Mortazavi et al. (2021) share the story of a 38 year old patient who, after undergoing 28 root canal restorations and 4 extractions with pain originating in the left premolar region and radiating to the contralateral mandibular region, neck, head and shoulders, was referred to the maxillofacial surgeon diagnosed as atypical odontalgia and treated with fluoxetine and clonazepam (11).

In this study, according to NT and age, there is a mean ratio of 41.7% in the age range 41-60 and 61-80 years, followed by 12.6% in the age range 20-40 years and 3.9% between 81-95 years of age; especially in the latter age group, there are clinical data of patients who have died at the present time, perhaps due to natural causes or the COVID-19 virus, the results of which are also reflected in the literature; by virtue of the fact that young people, more females than males in a 3 to 1 ratio, under 40 years of age suffering from TN, may be a first symptom of multiple sclerosis; a finding distinguished in patients seen in EsSalud Cusco from January 2019 to August 2022.

On the influence of gender, at the national level: First of all Tragodara (2020), if not treated adequately, it can lead to stress at work, social, psychological and even suicide (17). Secondly, Vasquez (2020), it is more common in females at 76.7%, with the V2 branch being mostly affected at 33.23% (14). In the international arena: With another perspective Boto (2010), according to some authors it is more frequent in males (1.2:1) and for others more in women. Its incidence is 4 per 100,000 inhabitants and generally affects the right hemiarch to 60% of cases, 39% is manifested on the left side *and 1% bilaterally with appearances of alternating pain especially in cases of multiple sclerosis* (5). Furthermore, according to Von Eckardstein and Veit Rohde (2015), TN is often triggered by chewing and manipulation of the gums. Therefore, patients are likely to consult their dentist when it first presents before being referred to a neurologist or neurosurgeon. As an example, of 51 patients; two-thirds reported being pain free; forty-one patients (82%) initially consulted their dentist; of these, 27 received invasive dental treatment for pain syndrome, including extractions, root canals and implants. Differential diagnoses include odontogenic pain syndromes, as well as atypical orofacial pain; summing up that the current literature recognises the difficulties in correctly diagnosing trigeminal neuralgia (3). Along the same lines, Alcantara and Gonzales (2017), the American Academy of Neurology (AAN), developed a new taxonomy with diagnostic accuracy criteria, with a classification system for neuropathic pain, created to be applied in diagnostic and treatment decisions (19). In fact, Gossweiler (2018), this case report describes the application of major autohaemotherapy, 3 sessions for 14 days prior to exodontia of tooth 36 to facilitate resolution of TN, with no symptomatology at 4 months follow-up, as a result of a chronic dental infection in that tooth in a female patient (20). In addition, Grin et al. (2018), through a complete examination including CT, MRI and laboratory, avoid entering the root canal of affected teeth and proceed to the pharmacological intake of carbamazepine. It should not be forgotten that this pathology presents as odontogenic pain, which is why it is urgent for stomatologists to be aware of its symptoms (13). Likewise, Antonaci et al. (2020), recruited 102 patients, mostly women with an F:M ratio of 2.64:1 (1). In contrast, Ayele et al. (2020), 50.8% of whom were male, 41% had a history of dental extractions on the involved side; a well-defined trigger zone was identified in one third (36%) of cases. Carbamazepine was the most prescribed drug with a median dose of 600 mg (RIQ: 400 - 1000 mg). In conclusion, a statistically significant number of patients with single-branch involvement reported outstanding satisfaction with their treatment compared to those with multi-branch involvement (95% CI: 1.3-3.8: p = 0.006) (8). According to De Laat (2020), in order not to confuse odontogenic pain with non-odontogenic pain (myofascial, trigeminal neuropathy, as well as painful post-traumatic trigeminal neuropathic pain, orofacial neurovascular pain, cardiac and paranasal sinus disease), a good systematic HC with adequate anamnesis, detailed dental, periodontal and intraoral examination and a general orofacial radiography are necessary (21). In this regard, Jaramillo and Mendoza (2020), in their study, 67% of the participants were 26 females and 33% were 13 males (22). In this regard, Tripathi et al. (2020), out of 187 patients, only 117 participated, whereby about 55.5% of the patients had odontalgia and 65.8% of them visited a dentist. About 41.8% of patients underwent a dental procedure; 18.8% had worsening pain, while 8.5% had some partial improvement. About 19.6% also underwent root canal treatment, while 6.8% had a nerve block. An average of 1.6 teeth were extracted per person. 71 % of patients were satisfied with gamma-knife radiosurgery for TN; therefore, there is a need for a better understanding of the disease among dentists and patients for timely and correct treatment without undergoing extractions. Therefore, the onus is on neurosurgeons/neurologists to disseminate knowledge about proper diagnosis and treatment modalities (10). As for Bara et al. (2021), as a treatment, carbamazepine has some anticholinergic effects; discovered in 1962 it changed the natural history of the disease; four years later it was marketed as Tegretol, with enthusiastic results. Of course, surgery has made remarkable advances: Janetta's microvascular decompression, focusing on Gasser's ganglion, from the hypotheses of demyelination to the "switching on" of models due to injured and hyperexcitable axons (23). Thus Duran and Duran (2021), out of 5070 neurological patients, 3280 were female (64.7%) and 1790 were male (35.3%); 151 were female (2.97%), 86 were male (1.69%). Forty-one percent had CNS involvement (headache, vertigo, convulsions, memory disorders, tremor), 57% PNS involvement (paraesthesia, weakness, painful polyneuropathy, trigeminal neuralgia), 45% musculoskeletal involvement (myalgia, polyarthralgia) and 35% neuropsychiatric involvement (anxiety, depression, insomnia). The majority (78%) had 2 to 4 symptoms. 24). According to Inoyatova et al. (2021), the most affected side of the face is the right (60%), and to a lesser extent the left; but simultaneous bilateral pain in TN is rare (1.7%-5%). However, these patients frequently experience paroxysms of unilateral alternating lateral pain. In terms of pain, the maxillary (V2) and mandibular (V3) branches are most commonly involved, although a quarter of cases affect the ophthalmic division (V1). Thus: Only V2 (32.5%), V2 and V3 (42.5%) on the right side of the process (53%), with a predominance of women (64.8%). On the basis of the data obtained, it was shown that the intensity of the pain syndrome can be judged by means of the Beck Depression Scale and the VAS. The Beck Depression Scale in this study does not reflect an objective picture of acute pain syndrome, especially in the comparison group (25). In contrast, Kaya and Kaya (2021), in a clinical report, although the dental radiograph was normal, amoxicillin/clavulanic acid (2x1 g daily) was administered. After the use of the first dose of antibiotic, he developed angioedema and his general condition worsened. Methylprednisolone 80 mg intravenously was administered in the emergency department. With this treatment, all ailments recovered, including facial, mandibular and dental pain (9). According to Lara C. (2021), it is generally caused by compression of vessels on the nerve, but there are exceptions, where this condition does not develop, with 4-13 cases per 100,000 inhabitants and above all in the female public (26). On the other hand, Maarbjerg and Benoliel (2021), the new International Classification of Headache Disorders (ICHD) for TN is based on reliable clinical data, imaging and neurophysiological studies. Therefore, further research is needed on the associated clinical signs (lacrimation and sensory changes), as well as on all aspects of TN (natural history, clinical picture, diagnosis, treatment and prognosis); with emphasis on rigorous investigations of surgical alternatives for the different subtypes of TN and improved pharmacotherapy (2). In that framework Mo et al. (2021), TN is associated with a distinctive whole brain structural neuroimaging pattern to differentiate between morphological phenotypes, (12). According to Mortazavi et al. (2021), announcing the report of a man with atypical odontalgia (OA), dentists should consider the visual analogue scale (VAS) when confronted with odontalgia without a reasonable organic cause to avoid unnecessary dental procedures (11). In that Slettebo (2021), of 102 patients who consulted for facial pain, 38 patients were first referred to a neurologist, 1 patient to a neurosurgeon and 1 patient to an oral surgeon for surgical treatment of the suspected TN. All these 38 patients had been examined by one or more dentists before consulting their neurologist. Therefore, misdiagnosis is a major factor against health, as patients may face unnecessary risks and futile neurosurgery, in addition to delayed treatment of their underlying painful condition (27). In this regard, Abril et al. (2022), by developing a correct clinical history with adequate complementary examinations, the diagnosis is correct and a lack of information about TN is prevented, preventing dentists and endodontists from unfounded root canal treatment. Therefore, the mastery and knowledge of this pathophysiology would be of particular help to stomatologists and endodontists. Likewise, neurologists and neurosurgeons could differentiate typical and atypical TN from odontogenic pain (28). Chen et al. (2022) point out that most patients present with a normal physical and neurological examination, in which reliable biomarkers for the disease are lacking (29). Finally Jay and Barkin (2022), The International Classification of Headache Disorders, Edition 3 (ICHD-3), suggests: recurrent paroxysms of unilateral facial pain in the distribution of one or more divisions of the trigeminal nerve, lasting a fraction of a second to two minutes, severe and electric shock-like, stabbing, or sharp stabbing and may be precipitated by innocuous stimuli both with and without the affected trigeminal dermatome. Therefore, a thorough history and neurological examination are essential to achieve the correct diagnosis (4).

In this research, as far as NT and sex are concerned, it discovers an average relationship, with 79.5% or 100 females, compared to the male sector of 20.5% or 27 males; both in the years 2019 at 6.3%, 2020 at 44.1%, 2021 at 35.4% and 2022 for 14.2%; the sharp increase from 2019 to 2020 as a possible psychological effect due to the COVID 2019 pandemic, and its progressive decrease in cases to 2022. Therefore, this aetiology becomes the most prevalent of all, as indicated by most of the literature and the INEI in the national population in 2020 according to sex.

In reference to the year, the research background on NT, shows in plurality the period 2020 and 2021 as follows: in the Peruvian territory both Tragodara (2020) and Vasquez (2020); at the international level Antonaci et al. (2020), Ayele et al.

(2020), De Laat (2020), Jaramillo and Mendoza (2020), Tripathi et al. (2020), Bara et al. (2021), Duran and Duran (2021), Inoyatova et al. (2021), Kaya and Kaya (2021), Lara C. (2021), Maarbjerg and Benoliel (2021), Mannerak et al. (2021), Maarbjerg and Benoliel (2021), Mannerak et al. (2021), Mo et al. (2021), Molina et al. (2021), Mortazavi et al. (2021), Slettebo (2021), Smith et al. (2021).

In the present research for the year 2022, the casuism is as follows: In 2019 6.3%, in

2020 44.1%, in 2021 35.4% and in 2022 14.2%; consistent with the studies and with the outcome of COVID 19, in positive tests and side effects post COVID vaccine.
In the field of COVID: Firstly, Duran and Duran (2021), for a report 237 patients presented with post-COVID neurological manifestations (4.67%). Therefore, "post-COVID neurological syndrome" represents a diagnostic challenge for the clinical neurologist because of the multiple manifestations: central and peripheral nervous system, with musculoskeletal and neuropsychiatric symptoms, without a classic semiology, with intense and constant headache, overuse, insomnia, anxiety and unexplained depression in patients with no history of COVID. 24). Second, Kaya and Kaya (2021); a patient developed acute trigeminal neuritis after Pfizer-BioNTech's SARS-CoV-2 vaccine and at the same time, the patient was consulted for toothache (9). Subsequently Molina et al. (2021), although the PCR test was negative, for the 65-year-old patient, the rapid test showed positive IgM and IgG serology for SARS-CoV-2, and an initial analysis showed a slightly elevated D-dimer of 800 ng/ml (upper limit: 500 ng/ml). Due to these findings, the patient was diagnosed with TN secondary to SARS-CoV-2 viral infection. However, the pain resolved with the improvement of COVID- 19 specific symptoms. Therefore, the new SARS-CoV-2 coronavirus is a possible aetiology of secondary TN. However, further studies are needed to elucidate the neuropathology of this viral infection (16).
Regarding TN and COVID, this survey likewise states an average relationship in patients seen at the Hospital Adolfo Guevara Velasco, from January 2019 to August 2022; through which 3.1% of patients diagnosed with TN, revealed a positive test for COVID 19, responding to the type of secondary TN; while 1.6% tested negative.In reference to vaccinations, 1.6% of patients were vaccinated against COVID 19, of which one vaccinated patient reported being diagnosed with post-vaccination secondary TN; conversely, 1.6% of insured persons were not vaccinated; finally, 98.4% of patient data did not record such information. This is consistent with the scarce findings from other South American and European latitudes.
As for genetics: According to Boto (2010), it is rarely genetic (5). While Mannerak et al. (2021), about 1-2% of TN cases have a hereditary form. Available human studies propose the following genes as possible contributors to the development of TN: CACNA1A, CACNA1H, CACNA1F, KCNK1, TRAK1, SCN9A, SCN8A, SCN3A, SCN10A, SCN5A, NTRK1, GABRG1, MPZ gene, MAOA gene and SLC6A4. Thus, their role in familial TN remains to be addressed. In sum, this systematic review suggests a more important role of genetic factors in the pathogenesis of TN than previously assumed (7). Finally, Smith et al. (2021), researchers found multiple genetic and molecular targets involved in possible pathophysiologies that are related to the development of trigeminal neuralgia, demonstrating the possibility that the genetic predisposition to trigeminal neuralgia may involve multiple genes and/or downstream products, such as ion channels, thus TN may be multi-causal. For this reason, the inability of the neurovascular compression model to satisfactorily account for a significant subset of patients with sporadic and familial TN has led to the investigation

of alternative models, especially those involving ion channels (6).

In the present study, the NT and genetics theme developed a medium relationship, with a greater participation of cases of the mestizo Cuzco ethnic group, comprising 73.2% of the cases studied, as opposed to 26.8% of the purely indigenous ethnic group. Of these, it should be remembered that the majority are female, so the ethnic component, more than the genetics itself, is a factor to be taken into account. This is probably due to the mix of ethnic groups from different parts of the world, especially Spanish and African.

As for the tumour: To begin with Antonaci et al. (2020), there is an urgent need to increase neurological knowledge in order to recognise the clinical picture of TN in a timely manner and to adhere properly to specific guidelines. This may result in a favourable outcome for patients, whose quality of life is often severely affected (1). Next Mo et al. (2021), patients with trigeminal neuralgia (TN) exhibited reductions in cortical indices in the anterior cingulate cortex (ACC), medial cingulate cortex (MCC) and posterior cingulate cortex (PCC) relative to controls. In addition, they had a generalised reduction in subcortical volume that was most evident in the putamen, thalamus, accumbens, pallidum and hippocampus (12). Focusing on pharmacological treatment, Alcantara and Sanchez (2016), (carbamazepine 100mg- 2 times daily, Oxcarbazepine 300mg- 2 times daily, Baclofen 5mg- 3 times daily, gabapentin 100mg- 3 times daily, pregabalin 75mg one nightly intake, lamotrigine 25mg - once daily, phenytoin 50mg - 3 times daily, topiramate 25mg - a nightly dose for 7 days and then increase for 1-2 weeks in doses of 25-50mg twice daily, levetiracetam 250mg - twice daily); However, the non-resolution by medication leads to surgery, either open or conservative percutaneous, which is very effective, as well as radiofrequency thermocoagulation, which is 97% effective against pain, with a recurrence after half an anus of 25% and with the presence of pain after a decade of 52%.3%; as complications, facial hypoaesthesia 1-9% and corneal anaesthesia 0-17% (18).

In the present scientific investigation, the tumour and TN also reflect an average relationship, with 7.9% compatible with 10 people with the presence of a tumour case, 15 people corresponding to 11.8% who do not report a tumour case, and 80.3% of the data, comprising 102 patients, do not record any data in their medical records. Of this casuistry, some of these patients had to be submitted to the Neurosurgery service for surgery, given that only 6.3% were evaluated by means of nuclear magnetic resonance (NMR). On the other hand, this is the list of drugs and treatments used in neurology, neurosurgery and dentistry in EsSalud Cusco against trigeminal neuralgia in the 127 patients: Antineuralgics (fluoxetine 20mg, sertriline hydrochloride 50mg), antineuropatics (gabapentin 300mg, tricyclic antidepressant amitriptyline 25mg, carbamazepine 200mg, magnesium valproate 200mg, valproic acid 250mg, clonazepam 0.5mg, lamotrigine 50mg, oxcarbazepine 300mg, pregabalin 75mg), antidepressant neuromodulators (mirtazapine 30mg, venfalaxine 75mg, sulpiride 50 and 200mg), oral or intravenous analgesics; glucocorticoid (dexamethasone IM 8mg/2ml), opioids (paxelis 50mg, tramadol drops 100mg/ml and tramadol hydrochloride 100mg), NSAIDs (diclofenac 75mg/3ml, paracetamol 500mg, naproxen 250mg, indomethacin 25mg). Benzodiazepines (alprazolam 0.5mg), vitamin B1 (thiamine hydrochloride 300mg), multi-vitamin complex (neurobion 25000, pyridoxine hydrochloride 50mg), muscle relaxants (orphenadrine VIM 60mg/2ml), gastroprotectors (omeprazole 20mg, ranitidine 150mg) and radiological contrast agent (iohexol equivalent 350mg iodine/ml x 100ml). Overdose; acupuncture, botulinum toxin 1 ampoule/100U, cannabis drops 30ml, one cat drop 60x 300mg. Medication: Carbamazepine 200mg, Gabapentin 300mg, starting with low doses every 24 hours and according to the response, increasing the amount. As for neurosurgery: Surgery for trigeminal neuralgia, suboccipital craniectomy (with teflon between vessel and nerve with mild facial paralysis with physical medicine and rehabilitation therapy), craniotomy, trigeminal microvascular decompression, gamma knife and rhizotomy.

As far *as demyelination* is concerned*, according* to Lara C. (2021), according to Moses, Beaver and Kerr, according to research into radicular demyelination of the nerve, it is manifested by vascular compression of the posterior radicular region, with the presence of irregular degenerative myelin in the course of the trigeminal nerve and due to this segmental demyelination, non-synaptic transmissions are revealed, giving rise to triggers (26).

The demyelination in this research, by means of nuclear magnetic resonance (NMR) used in 18 patients, registered this condition in 6 patients; demonstrating that 89.8% did not register any data in their clinical record, while 4.7% did present it and 5.5% did not manifest it. Due to a factor external to the consultation, such as the failure and disuse of this medical equipment since 2020, only 18 patients out of the 127 analysed benefited, to the detriment of the rest; alternatively, 15 multi-slice spiral tomographies (TEM) and 13 computerised axial tomographies (TAC) were verified.

Jaramillo and Mendoza (2020), *because of its unknown cause, it is essential to have a specialist medical consultation to rule out systemic diseases such as diabetes and arterial hypertension* (22). According to Chen et al. (2022), the aetiology of TN is probably multifactorial in many patients; only a small percentage of patients with TN present with demonstrable compression or morphological changes in the trigeminal nerve, and neurovascular compression does not always translate into disease; fortunately, surgical and minimally invasive interventions seem to have a promising solution (29). Finally, Jay and Barkin (2022), isolated "facial migrane" is very rare (0.2%), triggering misdiagnosis with dental and maxillary sinus pathology (4).

To complete this analysis of the unknown aetiology, 26% of the 127 cases did not declare any record in the computerised medical data of EsSalud-Cusco, 55.1% highlighted the presence of this component and 18.9% did not fit into this problem, confirming the problem of the medical apparatus. Finally, with regard to pupillary dilation, 96.1% of the clinical data did not record any information, and only 3.9% indicated that they did not report it, as the experts did not attach any importance to ocular expression.

CONCLUSIONS

1. It was identified that the average ratio of the most common aetiology of trigeminal neuralgia has as a predisposing factor; sex, being female the most affected in a percentage of 79.5%; and as an aetiological factor, the unknown aetiology, manifested as the highest proportion at 55.1%, in patients seen in EsSalud Cusco from January 2019 to August 2022. The highest cases of TN were reported in 2020 at 44.1%, with lower casuistry in 2019 at 6.3%; probably due to the anxiety of the pandemic. In conclusion, demyelination cases only reflected 4.7% of the population studied.
2. It was found that there is a medium relationship between TN and age, especially between the ages of 41-80 years at 41.7%; according to Inoyatova, middle-aged and older patients suffer more often from TN at 66.7%. However, more young women under 40 years of age, in a range of 3 to 1, suffering from TN, could be a first symptom of multiple sclerosis.
3. It was found that there is an average relationship between TN and sex, being: 79.5% in women, more affected the left facial side in 35.4%; with a type of idiopathic TN in 34.6%; of an intense pain in 59.1% according to the VAS scale; above all, according to the Alcantara and Gonzalez pain test, the 3 branches V1, V2 and V3 were more affected in 18.9%; an abrupt onset of pain in 55.9%, lasting less than 2 minutes in 11%; a spontaneous type in 49.6%; whose stimulation was more mechanical than innocuous in 55.9%; whose pain between paroxysms was reflected in 11%; whose stimulation was more mechanical and innocuous in 55.9%; whose pain between paroxysms was reflected in 11%; whose pain between paroxysms was more mechanical than mechanical.9%, lasting less than 2 minutes in 11%; spontaneous type in 49.6%; whose stimulus was more innocuous mechanical in 55.9%; whose pain between paroxysms was reflected in 37.8%; with an additional continuous pain of 55.1% and manifesting grimaces in 5 patients at 3.9%, with a daily pain frequency of 29.9%; in short, no patient was referred to Lima.
4. It was found that there is an average relationship between NT and COVID in patients seen in EsSalud Cusco from January 2019 to August 2022; 3.1% of patients with NT revealed a positive COVID 19 test, responding to the type of secondary NT, while 1.6% tested negative. Regarding the vaccinated patients, both when receiving the anti-COVID vaccine and not receiving it, in both cases the statistical figures were equivalent to 1.6%; among them, a 51-year-old patient of indigenous ethnicity, vaccinated with the 4ª dose, declared to be diagnosed with secondary type TN, post-vaccination.
5. It was pointed out that there is an average relationship between genetics and TN, where one of the most outstanding points was the greater participation of findings found in the medical history data of the mestizo ethnic group, comprising 73.2% of the cases studied compared to 26.8% of the indigenous ethnic group. Of these, it should be remembered that the majority are female, so the ethnic component, more than the genetics itself, is a factor to be taken into consideration.
6. A mean relationship between tumour factor and TN was found to exist in 7.9% of

tumour cases; however, pupillary dilation was not present in 3.9% and was not recorded in 96.1% of the patients' medical data. Mostly, some of these patients had to undergo chirography by the neurosurgery department; however, only 18 patients underwent magnetic resonance imaging (MRI).

RECOMMENDATIONS

1. It is suggested that the dental profession should seek further consultation with Neurology in the event of diagnostic doubts in cases of atypical odontalgia, especially in female patients.
2. It is recommended that the specialties of Neurology and Neurosurgery, train and clarify the diagnosis of Trigeminal Neuralgia in the dental profession, even more so in age ranges over 40 years.
3. Dentists are advised to differentiate between electric shock pain and the throbbing pain characteristic of pulpitis, especially in female populations.
4. Dentists are invited to be familiar with the diagnosis of Trigeminal Neuralgia, in order to avoid extractions as well as unjustified root canals and these can be referred to the neurologist, considering a history of positive COVID and vaccinated patients.
5. The Colegio Odontologico del Peru is entrusted with the task of further disseminating Trigeminal Neuralgia among its members and the community in general, with special emphasis on care for the mestizo population.
6. It is recommended to the authorities of EsSalud, to include the diagnosis CIE G50.0 of Trigeminal Neuralgia in the area of Odontology; above all, to repair or acquire a new MRI, since we could be facing a tumour case.

BIBLIOGRAPHICAL REFERENCES

1 . Antonaci, F., Arceri, S., Rakusa, M., Mitsikostas, D. D., Milanov, I., Todorov, V., Ramusino, M. C., & Costa, A. Pitfalls in recognition and management of trigeminal neuralgia. Journal of Headache and Pain. 2020; 21(1): 1-8. doi: https://doi.org/10.1186/s10194- 020-01149-8

2 . Maarbjerg S, Benoliel R. The changing face of trigeminal neuralgia-A narrative review. HeadacheJournal. 2021 Jul; 61(6): 817-837. doi: https://doi.org/10.1111/head.14144

3 . Von Eckardstein KM, Veit Rohde MK. Unnecessary dental procedures as a consequence of trigeminal neuralgia.

4 . Jay G, Barkin R. Trigeminal neuralgia and persistent idiopathic facial pain (atypical facial pain). Science Direct. 2022 Jun; 68(6): doi: https ://doi.org/10.1016/j.disamonth.2021.101302

5 . Boto GR. Trigeminal neuralgia. Scielo. 2010 Oct; 21(5). Doi: Scielo.isciii.es/scielo.ph

6 . Smith CA, Paskhover B, Mammis A. Molecular mechanisms of trigeminal neuralgia: A systematic review. Science Direct. 2021 Jan; 200 (2021): 106397. doi https://doi.org/10.1016Zj.clineuro.2020.106397

7 . Mannerak MA, Lashkarivand A, Eide PK. Trigeminal neuralgia and genetics: A systematic review. Molecular Pain. 2021 jan. doi: 10.1177/17448069211016139

8 . Ayele, B A, Mengesha AT, Zewde YZ. Clinical characteristics and associated factors of trigeminal neuralgia: Experience from Addis Ababa, Ethiopia. BMC Oral Health. 2020; 20(1): 1-7. doi: https://doi.org/10.1186/s12903-020-01227- У

9 . Kaya A, Kaya SY. A case of trigeminal neuralgia developing after a COVID-19 vaccination. Journal of NeuroVirology. 2021 dec; 28(2022): 181-182. doi: https ://link. springer.com/ article/10.1007/s13365 -021-01030-7

10 Tripathi M, Sadashiva N, Gupta A, Jani P, Pulickal SJ, Deora H, Kaur R, Kaur P, Batish A, Mohindra S, Kumar N. Please spare my teeth! Dental procedures and trigeminal neuralgia. Surgical Neurology International. 2020 dec; 11(455): 1-5. doi: 10.25259/SNI_729_2020. eCollection 2020.

11 Mortazavi, H., Baharvand, M., Far, K. R., & Eznaveh, Z. S. (2021). Dental extraction and full mouth root canal therapy in a patient with atypical odontalgia: Report of invasive malpractice. BDS. 2021 Jan- mar; 24(1): 1-4. doi: https ://doi.org/10.14295/bds.2021.v24i1.2315

12 Mo J, Zhang J, Hu W, Luo F, Zhang K. Whole-brain morphological alterations associated with trigeminal neuralgia. J Headache Pain 22. 2021 aug; 95 (2021). doi: https://doi.org/10.1186/s10194-021-01308-5

13 . Grin EJ, Grin P, Rocha ML. Trigeminal neuralgia: a case report. Rev ADM. 2018; 75(3): 164-167. doi: https://www.medigraphic.com/pdfs/adm/od-2018/od183i.pdf.

14 Vasquez DA. Frequency of trigeminal neuralgia in patients treated at the National Hospital Almanzor Aguinaga Asenjo, Chiclayo, period 2010-2017. ALICIA. 2020.

15 Perez, M. (2019). Action research in teaching practice. *Javeriana*, 177-192. https://doi.org/10.11144/Javeriana.m12-24.ncev

16 Molina J, Gonzales L, Garcia C. Trigeminal neuralgia as the sole neurological manifestation of COVID-19: A case report. Headache journal. March 2021; 61 (3). doi: https://doi.org/10.1111/head.14075

17 Tragodara KM. Trigeminal neuralgia: a physiotherapeutic approach. ALICIA. 2020. http://repositorio.uigv.edu.pe/handle/20.500.11818/4932

18 Alcantara A, Sanchez C.I. Actualizacion em el manejo de la neuralgia del trigemino. ELSEVIER. 2016 May-Jun; 42(4):244-253. doi: 10.1016/j.semerg.2015.09.007

19 Alcantara A, Gonzales A. Trigeminal neuralgia: New classification and diagnostic classification for clinical practice and research. Scielo. 2017 Apr; 24(2). doi: https://dx.doi.org/10.20986/resed.2016.3483/2016

20 Gossweiler, AG. Case report Management of a patient with Trigeminal Neuralgia associated with failed endodontic therapy using Ozone Therapy : A Case Report. Spanish Journal of Ozone Therapy. 2018 May; 8(1): 129-143. doi: https://www.semanticscholar.org/paper/Management-of-a-patient-with- Trigeminal-Neuralgia-A- Gossweiler/50be77d80e9436b4cef414fa0303950acf1987d4

21 De Laat, A. Differential diagnosis of toothache to prevent erroneous and unnecessary dental treatment. Journal of Oral Rehabilitation. 2020 Jun; 47(6): 775-781. doi: https://doi.org/10.1111/joor. 12946

22 Jaramillo DE, Mendoza FA. Prevalence of trigeminal neuralgia in patients attended in the stomatology area of the Teodoro Maldonado Carbo Hospital. Bachelor Thesis. 2020 jun. http://repositorio.ug.edu.ec/handle/redug/48572

23 Bara S, Vyshka G, Ranxha E. A historical note on the treatment of trigeminal neuralgia. TOPAINJ. 2021 Oct; 14 (9-13). doi: 10.2174/1876386302114010009

24 Duran JC, Duran JP. Post COVID-19 neurological syndrome: A prospective study at 3600m above sea level in La Paz Bolivia.JNS. 2021 Oct; 429. doi:https://doi.org/10.1016/j.jns.2021.119820g

25 Inoyatova SO, Madjidova YN, Mukhammadsolikh. Clinical and Neurological Peculiarities of Trigeminal Neuralgia. IJMSCR. 2021 Sept; 01(07). Doi: https://doi.org/10.47191/ijmscrs/v1-i7-11

26 Lara C. Update on the management of Trigeminal Neuralgia. University of Seville. 2021 jun. https://hdl.handle.net/11441/134673

27 . Slettebo, H. (2021). Is this really trigeminal neuralgia ? Diagnostic re- evaluation of patients referred for neurosurgery. 2021 Oct; 21(4): 788-793. Scandinavian Journal of Pain. doi: https ://doi.org/10.1515/sjpain-2021-0045

28 Abril MC, Cardenas MF, Duarte AM. Trigeminal neuralgia as a determinant factor in the administration of unnecessary endodontic treatment. USTA Repository. 2022 Jun. doi: http://hdl.handle.net/11634/45320

29 Chen Q, Ik Yi D, Joco JN, Liu M, Chang SD, Barad MJ, Lim M, Qian X. The molecular basis and pathophysiology of trigeminal neuralgia. Int. J. Mol. Sci. Mar

2022; 23(7): 3604. doi: https://doi.org/10.3390/ijms23073604
30 Prasad G. Handbook of trigeminal neuralgia. Singapore: Springer; 2019.
31 Ballester, B. (2004). Bases metodologicas de la investigacion educativa. Palma de Mallorca.
32 Gallardo, Y., and Moreno, A. (1999). Recoleccion de la informacion. Santa Fe de Bogota.
https://academia.utp.edu.co/grupobasicoclmicayaplicadas/files/2013/06Z3.-Collecting-Information-LEARN-INFORMATION-LEARN-IN-APRENDER-IN-APPROACH
INVESTIGAR-ICFES.pdf
33 Gonzales, N., Zerpa, M., Gutierrez, D and Pirela C. (2007). La investigacion educativa en el hacer docente. *Laurus*, 13(23), 279-309. https ://www.redalyc.org/pdf/761/76102315 .pdf

ANNEXES

PROBLEMS	OBJECTIVES	HYPOTHESIS	VARIABLES
General problem	**Overall objective**	**General hypothesis**	**Variable Y**
i,What is /э *etiology mds common to* **the Neuralgia of the trigdmino at** patients attended at EsSalud Cusco since January 2019 until August 2022?	Identify *mds theology common to* **the Neuralgia of the trigdmino in** patients attended in EsSalud Cusco since January 2019until August 2022	There is a *mds etiology common to* the **Neuralgia of the trigdmino** in patients attended in EsSalud Cusco since January 2019until August 2022	**Neuralgiadel trigdmlno** - Cldsica - Secondary - Idiopathic - Pain
Problems Specific	**Objectives Specific**	**Hypothesis Specific**	**Variable X**
1) ^Exists relationship between the NT **y** *age* at patients attended at EsSalud Cusco from January 2019 to August 2022?	Determine the relationship that exists between the NT *y the age* in patients attended in EsSalud Cusco since January 2019until August 2022	There is a relationship between the NT y *the age* at patients attended in EsSalud Cusco since January 2019until August 2022	***Most common aetiology*** Factors predisposing factors - Age - Sexo Aetiological factors - COVID - Genetics - Tumours - Demyelination - Aetiology uncooked
2) iWhich relationship there is between the NT **y** *sex* at patients attended in EsSalud Cusco from January 2019 to August 2022?	Compare it relationship that exists between the NT y *el дёпеzо* en patients attended in EsSalud Cusco since January 2019until August 2022	There is a relationship between the NT y *the дёпеzо* at patients attended in EsSalud Cusco since January 2019until August 2022	-
3) iCuaiesla relationship	Associate the relationship that	There is a relationship between the NT y *the*	

existing	exists between the NT	*COVID* at
between the NT *y the CO VID* at patients attended in EsSalud Cusco from January 2019 to August	y *COVID* in patients attended in EsSalud Cusco since January 2019until August 2022	patients attended in EsSalud Cusco since January 2019until August 2022

2022?		
4) <j,Qud type of relationship there is between the NT y *the* *∂eпëHca* at patients attended in EsSalud Cusco from January 2019 until August 2022?	Establish the relationship that exists between the NT y *la ∂eпëHca* en patients attended in EsSalud Cusco since January 2019until August 2022	Relationship Exists between the NT y *the* *∂eпëHca* at patients attended in EsSalud Cusco since January 2019until August 2022
5) <i,Qu6 The relationship is guard between the NT y *the* *tumours* at patients attended in EsSalud Cusco from January 2019 to August 2022?	Describe it relationship that exists between the NT y *tumours* in patients attended in EsSalud Cusco since January 2019until August 2022	There is a relationship between the NT y *the* *tumours* at patients attended in EsSalud Cusco since January 2019until August 2022

Annex 2. Data collection sheet

<u>Trigeminal neuralgia (TN) assessment sheet</u>

MOST COMMON AETIOLOGY

PREDISPOSING FACTORS			
Age	Aho of patient admission to EsSalud-Cusco		
1	From 20 to 40 years old	Aho 2019	
2	From 41 to 60 years old	Aho 2020	
3	From 61 to 80 years old	Aho 2021	
4	From 81 to 99 years	Aho 2022	
Sex			
1	Male (M)		
2	Female (F)		

AETIOLOGICAL FACTORS			
Covid-19	Yes( )	No( )	NR( )
Positive test	Yes( )	No( )	NR( )
Negative test	Yes( )	No( )	NR( )
Vaccinated	Yes( )	No( )	NR( )
Unvaccinated	Yes( )	No( )	NR( )
Genetics o dtnia	Yes( )	No( )	NR( )
family	White ( ) Mestizo (	) Indigenous (	) Afro ( )
Tumour Cause	Yes( )	No( )	NR( )
Demyelination	Sf( )/ With NMR ( )		No ( )/No NMR ( ) NR ( )/NR MRI ( )
Etiology unknown	**Yes( )**	**No( )**	**NR ( )**

TRIGEMINAL NEURALGIA

TYPES OF TRIGEMINAL NEURALGIA		
Classical ( ) Secondary Idiopathic ( ) ( )		No Registration ( )
PAIN SCALES		
Visual scale analogue (VAS)		
Pain Mild PainModerate PainSevere Pain 1-3 ( ) 4-6 ( ) 7-10 ( )		No pain/NR 0( )
Scale for the mentally handicapped y other criteria		
Grimaces SI( ) NO( )		No Registra( )
Pupillary dilatation SI( ) NO( )		No Registra(
Referring to	Lima SI( ) NO( )	No Registra(J˙
Frequency of pain Daily ( ) Weekly ( ) pain		No Registration ( )
Pain test Alcantara y Gonzalez		
Affected branches	V1 V2 V3 V1A/2 V2/v3 V1/V2/V3 Does not Register ()()()()() ( ) ( )	
Affected side	RightLeftBoth ( ) ( ) ( )	No Registra (T
Onset of pain	Mild Moderate *Rough* ( ) ( ) ( )	No Register .( )
Duraddn	*1Sec. to 2 min.* greater than 2 minutes ( ) ( )	No Registration ( )
Type of pain	*Provoked* *Spontaneous* ( ) ( )	No Registration ( )
Stimulus triggered	None *Mechanical* *Movements* No Record *( ) harmless ( )( ) ( ) ( )*	
Pain between paroxysms	Yes( ) No( )	No Registration ( )
Additional pain continue	Yes ( ) No ( )	No Registration ( )

Annex 3. Acceptance сото Research Mentor

LETTER OF ACCEPTANCE AS RESEARCH TUTOR IN ESSALUD- CUSCO

I Dr. Victor Edwin Ore Montalvo, neurologist of the Hospital Nacional Adolfo Guevara Velasco-EsSalud Cusco, with C.M. 36493, accept to be "Tutor" of this research work entitled: "Etiologia mas comun de la neuralgia del trigemino en pacientes atendidos en EsSalud Cusco desde el 2017 hasta la fecha", de tipo retrospective, para que se pueda indagar en las áreas de Neurologia, Neurocirugia y Odontologia, lo concemiente a esta investigacion; en beneficio de los pacientes y del gremio odontologico.

Cusco 06 September 2022

Annex 4. Informed Consent

INFORMED CONSENT

- **Dr. Julio Cdsar Espinoza Latorre**

Director of the National Hospital Adolfo Guevara Velasco- EsSalud Cusco

- **Head doctors of the Neurology, Neurosurgery and Dentistry units** of the National Hospital Adolfo Guevara Velasco - EsSalud Cusco.

The purpose of this document is to inform you what is going to be done with the data obtained from this study entitled **"Etiologia m£s comun de la Neuralgia del trigdmino en pacientes atendidos en EsSalud Cusco desde el 2017 hasta la fecha".**

The most common aetiology of TN in patients treated in this hospital could be identified for prevention in the referral of patients in future cases, especially in the field of dentistry.

This publication will be available to health professionals, students, patients and those interested in the field of trigeminal neuralgia.

Finally, this scientific research will be published in indexed journals, especially the Universitas Odontoldgica Journal of the Pontificia Universidad Javeriana- Colombia; the scientific book will be published virtually by the Editorial Acad6mica Espanola (eae) and the physical book will be donated to the library of the Hospital Nacional Adolfo Guevara Velasco - EsSalud Cusco.

....

Mg. C.D. Juan Pablo Nino de Guzman Zamalloa
Principal Investigator

Annex 5. Authorisation to investigate

SOLICITO: AUTORIZACION PARA REALIZAR TRABAJO DE INVESTIGACION

DR: JULIO CESAR ESPINOZA DE LA TORRE
DIRECTOR DEL HOSPITAL NACIONAL ADOLFO GUEVARA VELASCO CUSCO

Yo **C.D. Mg: Juan Pablo Niño de Guzmán Zamalloa** me dirijo a UD. con el debido respeto que se merece, me presento y expongo lo siguiente:

Solicitarle AUTORIZACION PARA REALIZAR TRABAJOS DE INVESTIGACION SOBRE **"Etiología más común de la Neuralgia del trigémino en pacientes atendidos en EsSalud Cusco desde el 2017 hasta la fecha"**. Por esta razón le suplico, su comprensión y atienda a mi petición en forma positiva para realizar dicho trabajo de investigación.

POR LO EXPUESTO:
Ruego a UD. acceder a mi petición por ser legal
Cusco,

....
NOMBRE: Juan Pablo Nino de Guzmán Zamalloa
DNI N.°: 43097455
TELEFONO: 981919740

Annex 6

Cusco

DR. JULIO CESAR ESPINOZA DE LA TORRE
DIRECTOR DEL HOSPITAL NACIONAL ADOLFO GUEVARA VELASCO ESSALUD- CUSCO

De mi consideración

El jefe de la unidad de **Neurología Dr. Víctor Edwin Oré Montalvo**, del Establecimiento de Salud HOSPITAL NACIONAL ADOLFO GUEVARA VELASCO ESSALUD-CUSCO de la Red Asistencial Cusco, donde se ejecutará el estudio titulado **"Etiología más común de la Neuralgia del trigémino en pacientes atendidos en EsSalud Cusco desde el 2017 hasta la fecha"**, cuyo investigador principal responsable es **C.D. Mg: Juan Pablo Niño de guzmán Zamalloa**, tiene el agrado de dirigirse a usted para manifestarle mi visto bueno para que el proyecto señalado previamente se ejecute en el Departamento/ Servicio/Area de **Neurología, Neurocirugía y Odontología**

Este proyecto deberá contar con la evaluación de Comité Institucional de Ética en investigación y la aprobación correspondiente por su despacho antes de su ejecución.

Sin otro particular, quedo de usted.

Atentamente

JEFE DE LA UNIDAD DE NEUROLOGÍA

Annex 7. Licence to conduct a scientific study
Dr. Julio Cesar Espinoza Latorre
Director of the National Hospital Adolfo Guevara Velasco- EsSalud Cusco
Request: To conduct a research study "Most common aetiology of trigeminal neuralgia in patients treated in EsSalud Cusco from January 2019 to August 2022".

First of all, with **the desire to contribute to improve the aetiology and dental care** of patients suffering from trigeminal neuralgia (TN), as they are seen by dentists and endodontists in daily practice, we frequently evaluate patients with this disease. This pathology should be seen in conjunction with neurology and neurosurgery. The present study will be carried out because cases of trigeminal neuralgia are presented in dental consultations and end up being treated by dentists (extractions) and/or endodontists (root canal treatment), when in fact they should be referred to the neurologist and according to the literature the COVID would also trigger this pathology. **It is intended to conduct a scientific research entitled: "Etiology most common trigeminal neuralgia in patients treated in EsSalud Cusco from 2017 to date", retrospective type,** in the areas of Neurology, Neurosurgery and Dentistry; finally, as suggested by the Neurologist Dr. Victor Edwin Ore Montalvo, this study should be conducted in this public institution and not in a private one because they have the exact data to 100% and free of bias. **Those working on this research, Cusquenian professionals and a Colombian**: *The former president of the Peruvian Society of Neurology and former neurologist of the National Hospital of EsSalud Edgardo Rebagliati Martins-Lima,* **Dr. Oscar Francisco Gonzales Gamarra, C.M 9059,** the future Master in Epidemiology in Washington DC- USA **C.D. Iriana Pena Manrique C.O.P. 28502,** the endodontist graduated at the Pontificia Universidad Javeriana **Nicolas Leon Perez C.O.C. 1026276991** and the expert in the field of endodontics for more than 10 years with internship at the Pontificia Universidad Javeriana-Colombia, with private clinical practice in Peru and Colombia **C.D. Juan Pablo Nino de Guzman Zamalloa C.O.P. 23413.**

To begin with, **it could be seen that there are few scientific investigations worldwide and only 2 updated investigations in Peru**. That is why, the interest was awakened to carry out a study focused on this area, due to complaints of apparently unresolved dental pain by the dental office. On the other hand, in evaluation, most of **the patients present normal physical and neurological examination, no biomarkers are found for this disease, so that research in all aspects and mainly the etiology is of great interest.** In view of the fact that the diagnosis is often an important factor in the solution of the pain presented by the patient during the dental consultation. Therefore, in the present study the different aetiologies will be evaluated in order to be referred to the respective speciality. Consequently, the incidence per year is estimated to be 4 persons per 100,000 inhabitants.

AN EXO 8

Cusco,

DR. JULIO CESAR ESPINOZA DE LA TORRE

DIRECTOR OF THE NATIONAL HOSPITAL ADOLFO GUEVARA VELASCO ESSALUD- CUSCO

Present.

Subject: Request for assessment and approval of research protocol

Of my own accord:

It is my pleasure to cordially greet you and request the evaluation of the research protocol entitled **"The most common aetiology of trigdminal neuralgia in patients treated in EsSalud Cusco from 2017 to date",** by the Research Committee and the Institutional Committee of £ Ethics in Research, as well as the presentation to the management for approval.

This is an observational study/clinical trial whose investigator mainly belongs to the **dental profession** in the Department/Service/Area of **Endodontics** of **exclusive private practice in Peru and Colombia. The** project will be carried out in the Research Centre/Department/Area **Neurology, Neurosurgery and Dentistry** of the National Hospital Adolfo Guevara Velasco ESSALUD of the Prestational/Asistential Network Cusco.

I would like to take this opportunity to renew to you the assurances of my highest consideration.

Yours sincerely,

....

NOMBRE: Juan Pablo Nino de Guzmán Zamalloa
DNI: 43097455
CELULAR: 981919740
CORREO: juanpablongz@gmail.com

NAME: Juan Pablo Nino de GuzrnAn Zamalloa
DNI: 43097455
CELLULAR: 981919740
MAIL: juanpablongz@gmail.com

Annex 9. Authorisation for research in Neurology, Neurosurgery and Dentistry units.

Dr. Victor Edwin Orë Montalvo

Neur6logo del Hospital Nacional Adolfo Guevara Velasco- EsSalud Cusco Request: Conduct a research study "Etiologia mas comun de la neuralgia del trigemino en pacientes atendidos en EsSalud Cusco desde enero del 2019 hasta agosto del 2022".

First and foremost, with the desire to contribute to improving the aetiology and dental care of patients suffering from trigeminal neuralgia (TN), as they are seen by dentists and endodontists in daily practice, we frequently evaluate patients with this disease. This pathology should be seen in conjunction with the neurology and neurosurgery areas. The present study will be carried out because cases of trigeminal neuralgia are presented in dental consultations and end up being treated by dentists (extractions) and/or endodontists (root canal treatment), when in fact they should be referred to neurologists and, according to the COVID literature, would also trigger this pathology. It is intended to conduct a scientific research entitled: "Etiologia most common trigdmino Neuralgia in patients treated in EsSalud Cusco from 2017 to date", retrospective type, in the areas of Neurology, Neurosurgery and Dentistry; finally. Those who work in this research, professionals cusquenos y a Colombian: *Ex presidents of the Peruvian Society of Neurology y ex Neurdlogo of the National Hospital of EsSalud Edgardo Rebagliati Martins- Lima,* Dr. Oscar Francisco Gonz&les Gamarra, C.M 9059, the future Magister in Epidemiology in Washington DC- USA C.D. Iriana Pena Manrique C.O.P. 28502, the endodontist graduated at the Pontificia Universidad Javeriana Nicolas Leon P6rez C.O.C. 1026276991 and the expert in the field of endodontics for more than 10 years with internship at the Pontificia Universidad Javeriana-Colombia, with private clinical practice in Peru and Colombia C.D. Juan Pablo Nino de Guzmin Zamalloa C.O.P. 23413.

To begin with, it could be seen that there are few scientific investigations at world level and only 2 updated investigations at the Peruvian level. For this reason, we decided to carry out a study focused on this area, due to complaints of apparently unresolved dental pain from the dental office. On the other hand, in evaluation, most of the patients have a normal physical and neurological examination, no biomarkers are found for this disease, so that research in all aspects and mainly the aetiology would be of great interest. In view of the fact that the diagnosis is often an important factor in the solution of the pain presented by the patient during the dental consultation. Therefore, in the present study the different aetiologies will be evaluated in order to be referred to the respective speciality. Consequently, сото incidence per year is estimated at 4 affected persons per 100000 inhabitants.

That is why we decided to appoint you as the "Tutor" of this research project, in order to develop it in this public institution EsSalud Cusco and not in a private one, since we have 100% accurate data free of bias.

Annex 10. Licence to conduct research and publish in an international indexed journal.
Dr. Julio Cesar Espinoza Latorre
Director of the National Hospital Adolfo Guevara Velasco- EsSalud Cusco
Request: To develop a study for an indexed international scientific journal on "The most common etiology of trigdminal neuralgia in patients treated in EsSalud Cusco from January 2019 to August 2022".

In order to be able to enhance and contribute to Peruvian research and make it better known internationally and in this sense, to improve the level of care for patients in the services of Dentistry, Neurology and Neurosurgery. It was decided to carry out an investigation on the **"Most common etiology of trigdminal neuralgia in patients treated in EsSalud Cusco from 2017 to date", to be published in the journal Universitas Odontologica of the Pontificia Universidad Javeriana de Colombia,** since **the researchers participating in this study both from Dentistry and Neurology,** we joined on this occasion to converge in the discipline of research, and in this way to serve the community and make this country a better place.

....

Principal Investigator
C.D. Juan Pablo Nino de Guzman Zamalloa
C.O.P. 23413
ID NO.: 43097455
TELEPHONE: 981919740

Annex 11. Resolution favourable to the management of the Cusco health care network of EsSalud

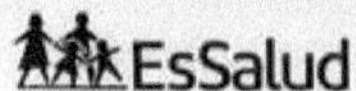

"Año del Fortalecimiento de la Soberanía Nacional"
"Decenio de la Igualdad de Oportunidades para Mujeres y Hombres"

RESOLUCION DE GERENCIA RED ASISTENCIAL CUSCO Nº 564-GRACU-ESSALUD-2022

CUSCO, 04 OCT 2022

VISTO,

La Nota de la Oficina de Capacitación, Investigación y Docencia Nº 397-OCID-GRACU-ESSALUD-2022 de fecha 28 de setembre de 2022, sobre la solicitud de emisión de la resolución de autorización de ejecución de Proyecto de Investigación;

CONSIDERANDO:

Que, mediante Resolución del Instituto de Evaluación de Tecnologías en Salud e Investigación Nº 46-IETSI-ESSALUD-2019 de fecha 03 de junio del 2019, se resuelve aprobar la Directiva Nº 003-IETSI-ESSALUD-2019 V.01 "Directiva que Regula el Desarrollo de la Investigación en Salud", cuyo objetivo es establecer los lineamientos para la aprobación, ejecución, supervisión, difusión, priorización y promoción de las actividades y estudios de investigación en salud a ser desarrollados en EsSalud.

Que, en el numeral 1 del Capítulo III – Disposiciones Generales de la Directiva Nº 003-IETSI-ESSALUD-2019 V.01, se establece que, la distinción entre ensayos clínicos y estudios observacionales se realiza según la definición regulatoria de ensayo clínico contenida en el Reglamento de Ensayos Clínicos y en esta Directiva, la misma que necesariamente corresponde a la definición metodológica. Los estudios que no cumplan la definición regulatoria de ensayo clínico serán considerados como estudios observacionales.

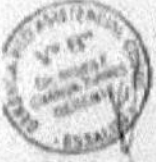

Que, en el numeral 2.1.1. de la Directiva Nº 003-IETSI-ESSALUD-2019 V.01, se establece que, los estudios observacionales se desarrollan mediante las siguientes modalidades: INSTITUCIONAL, EXTRA INSTITUCIONAL, COLABORATIVA Y TESIS DE PREGRADO;

Que, en el numeral 2.2.1 de la Directiva Nº 003-IETSI-ESSALUD-2019 V.01, se establece el proceso de aprobación de los estudios observacionales y la presentación de los documentos por parte del investigador principal (IP) o el coinvestigador responsable ante la Instancia Encargada del Área de Investigación (IEAI);

Que, en el numeral 2.2.2 de la Directiva Nº 003-IETSI-ESSALUD-2019 V.01, se establece que, la IEAI recibe el expediente y verifica el cumplimiento de los requisitos. Luego, envía el expediente al Comité Institucional de Ética en Investigación (CIEI) en un plazo que no exceda de tres días útiles;

Que, en el numeral 2.2.5 de la Directiva Nº 003-IETSI-ESSALUD-2019 V.01, se establece que, una vez aprobado el protocolo por el CIEI, la Gerencia evalúa el expediente y emite una carta dirigida al investigador con su decisión de autorizar o no el inicio del estudio en un plazo no mayor a catorce días calendario. La IEAI comunica la decisión al Comité y al IP haciéndole llegar la carta o certificado de aprobación del comité y de la gerencia. El Gerente del Órgano puede delegar esta función de autorización de estudios observacionales a otra instancia que considere conveniente, por ejemplo, a la IEAI o al director del establecimiento;

Que, mediante Resolución de Gerencia de Red Asistencial Cusco Nº 305-GRACU-ESSALUD-2020 de fecha 21 de setiembre del 2020 y su modificatoria con Resolución Nº 329-GRACU-ESSALUD-2020 de fecha 08 de octubre del 2020, se resuelve, conformar, a partir de la fecha y por el periodo de tres (03) años, el Comité Institucional de Ética en Investigación (CIEI) de la Gerencia de Red Asistencial Cusco del Seguro Social de Salud "ESSALUD".

//

www.essalud.gob.pe | Av. Anselmo Álvarez s/n
Wanchaq
Cusco, Perú
Telf.: 084-582890 y 084-228428

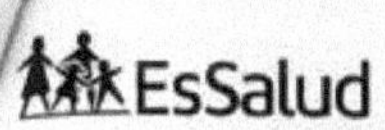

"Año del Fortalecimiento de la Soberanía Nacional"
"Decenio de la Igualdad de Oportunidades para Mujeres y Hombres"

Il. 2

RESOLUCION DE GERENCIA RED ASISTENCIAL CUSCO N° 564 -GRACU-ESSALUD-2022

Que, mediante documento del visto, la Oficina de Capacitación, Investigación y Docencia, en uso de sus atribuciones ha verificado el cumplimiento de los requisitos del Proyecto de Investigación con el Título "ETIOLOGÍA MÁS COMÚN DE LA NEURALGIA DEL TRIGÉMINO EN PACIENTES ATENDIDOS EN ESSALUD CUSCO DESDE EL 2017 HASTA LA FECHA", presentado por investigador principal Cirujano Dentista JUAN PABLO NIÑO DE GUZMAN ZAMALLOA. Dicho proyecto de investigación, entre otros cuenta con la aprobación del Comité de Ética en Investigación con Nota N° 62-CE-GRACU-ESSALUD-2022 de fecha 28 de setiembre de 2022; asimismo, cuenta con la opinión favorable de la sede donde se realizará la investigación según Anexo 6 suscrito por el Jefe de la Unidad de Neurología del Hospital Nacional "Adolfo Guevara Velasco" Doctor Victor Oré Montalvo;

Que, estando a los considerandos expuestos y en uso de las facultades conferidas mediante Directiva N° 003-IETSI-ESSALUD-2019 V.01 y Resolución de Presidencia Ejecutiva N° 67-PE-ESSALUD-2022.

SE RESUELVE:

PRIMERO.- **AUTORIZAR** la ejecución del Proyecto de Investigación con el Título **"ETIOLOGÍA MÁS COMÚN DE LA NEURALGIA DEL TRIGÉMINO EN PACIENTES ATENDIDOS EN ESSALUD CUSCO DESDE EL 2017 HASTA LA FECHA"**, presentado por investigador principal Cirujano Dentista JUAN PABLO NIÑO DE GUZMAN ZAMALLOA, a realizarse en los servicios de Neurología, Neurocirugía y Odontología del Hospital Nacional "Adolfo Guevara Velasco" de EsSalud Cusco.

SEGUNDO.- **DISPONER** que el investigador principal **JUAN PABLO NIÑO DE GUZMAN ZAMALLOA** prosiga con todas las acciones vinculadas con el tema de investigación, las cuales deberán ajustarse al cumplimiento de las normas y directivas de la institución establecidas para tal fin.

TERCERO.- **DISPONER** que las instancias respectivas brinden las facilidades del caso para la ejecución del Proyecto de Investigación autorizado con la presente Resolución.

REGÍSTRESE Y COMUNÍQUESE.

DR. RUBEN E. CRAHUA TORRES
CMP 34431 RNE 10018
RED ASISTENCIAL CUSCO
GERENTE
EsSalud

RECHT/aoq
Cc. OCID, CE, DHNAGV, INVESTIGADOR PRINCIPAL, ARCH.

1307	2022	4919

www.essalud.gob.pe

Av. Anselmo Álvarez s/n
Wanchaq
Cusco, Perú
Tel.: 084-582890 y 084-229428

Anexo 12 . Validación de los instrumentos para las variable X: Etiología más común y variable Y: Neuralgia de trigémino por expertos

"Etiología más común de la Neuralgia del trigémino en pacientes atendidos en EsSalud Cusco desde enero del 2019 hasta agosto del 2022".

Tabla 7
Validación de expertos

N.°	EXPERTOS	VARIABLE X	VARIABLE Y
1	Dr. Victor Edwin Oré Montalvo	100 %	
2	C.D. Soto Vidal Pedro Soto Santacruz	100 %	
3	Dr. Oscar Francisco Gonzáles Gamarra		100.00%
Total		%	%

Annex 13. Chi-Square X2 Distribution Table

P = Probabilidad de encontrar un valor mayor o igual que el chi cuadrado tabulado, v = Grados de Libertad

v/p	0,001	0,0025	0,005	0,01	0,025	0,05	0,1	0,15	0,2	0,25	0,3	0,35	0,4	0,45	0,5
1	10,8274	9,1404	7,8794	6,6349	5,0239	3,8415	2,7055	2,0722	1,6424	1,3233	1,0742	0,8735	0,7083	0,5707	0,4549
2	13,8150	11,9827	10,5965	9,2104	7,3778	5,9915	4,6052	3,7942	3,2189	2,7726	2,4079	2,0996	1,8326	1,5970	1,3863
3	16,2660	14,3202	12,8381	11,3449	9,3484	7,8147	6,2514	5,3170	4,6416	4,1083	3,6649	3,2831	2,9462	2,6430	2,3660
4	18,4662	16,4238	14,8602	13,2767	11,1433	9,4877	7,7794	6,7449	5,9886	5,3853	4,8784	4,4377	4,0446	3,6871	3,3567
5	20,5147	18,3854	16,7496	15,0863	12,8325	11,0705	9,2363	8,1152	7,2893	6,6257	6,0644	5,5731	5,1319	4,7278	4,3515
6	22,4575	20,2491	18,5475	16,8119	14,4494	12,5916	10,6446	9,4461	8,5581	7,8408	7,2311	6,6948	6,2108	5,7652	5,3481
7	24,3213	22,0402	20,2777	18,4753	16,0128	14,0671	12,0170	10,7479	9,8032	9,0371	8,3834	7,8061	7,2832	6,8000	6,3458
8	26,1239	23,7742	21,9549	20,0902	17,5345	15,5073	13,3616	12,0271	11,0301	10,2189	9,5245	8,9094	8,3505	7,8325	7,3441
9	27,8767	25,4625	23,5893	21,6660	19,0228	16,9190	14,6837	13,2880	12,2421	11,3887	10,6564	10,0060	9,4136	8,8632	8,3428
10	29,5879	27,1119	25,1881	23,2093	20,4832	18,3070	15,9872	14,5339	13,4420	12,5489	11,7807	11,0971	10,4732	9,8922	9,3418
11	31,2635	28,7291	26,7569	24,7250	21,9200	19,6752	17,2750	15,7671	14,6314	13,7007	12,8987	12,1836	11,5298	10,9199	10,3410
12	32,9092	30,3182	28,2997	26,2170	23,3367	21,0261	18,5493	16,9893	15,8120	14,8454	14,0111	13,2661	12,5838	11,9463	11,3403
13	34,5274	31,8830	29,8193	27,6882	24,7356	22,3620	19,8119	18,2020	16,9848	15,9839	15,1187	14,3451	13,6356	12,9717	12,3398
14	36,1239	33,4262	31,3194	29,1412	26,1189	23,6848	21,0641	19,4062	18,1508	17,1169	16,2221	15,4209	14,6853	13,9961	13,3393
15	37,6978	34,9494	32,8015	30,5780	27,4884	24,9958	22,3071	20,6030	19,3107	18,2451	17,3217	16,4940	15,7332	15,0197	14,3389
16	39,2518	36,4555	34,2671	31,9999	28,8453	26,2962	23,5418	21,7931	20,4651	19,3689	18,4179	17,5646	16,7795	16,0425	15,3385
17	40,7911	37,9462	35,7184	33,4087	30,1910	27,5871	24,7690	22,9770	21,6146	20,4887	19,5110	18,6330	17,8244	17,0646	16,3382
18	42,3119	39,4220	37,1564	34,8052	31,5264	28,8693	25,9894	24,1555	22,7595	21,6049	20,6014	19,6993	18,8679	18,0860	17,3379
19	43,8194	40,8847	38,5821	36,1908	32,8523	30,1435	27,2036	25,3289	23,9004	22,7178	21,6891	20,7638	19,9102	19,1069	18,3376
20	45,3142	42,3358	39,9969	37,5663	34,1696	31,4104	28,4120	26,4976	25,0375	23,8277	22,7745	21,8265	20,9514	20,1272	19,3374
21	46,7963	43,7749	41,4009	38,9322	35,4789	32,6706	29,6151	27,6620	26,1711	24,9348	23,8578	22,8876	21,9915	21,1470	20,3372
22	48,2676	45,2041	42,7957	40,2894	36,7807	33,9245	30,8133	28,8224	27,3015	26,0393	24,9390	23,9473	23,0307	22,1663	21,3370
23	49,7276	46,6231	44,1814	41,6383	38,0756	35,1725	32,0069	29,9792	28,4288	27,1413	26,0184	25,0055	24,0689	23,1852	22,3369
24	51,1790	48,0336	45,5584	42,9798	39,3641	36,4150	33,1962	31,1325	29,5533	28,2412	27,0960	26,0625	25,1064	24,2037	23,3367
25	52,6187	49,4351	46,9280	44,3140	40,6465	37,6525	34,3816	32,2825	30,6752	29,3388	28,1719	27,1183	26,1430	25,2218	24,3366
26	54,0511	50,8291	48,2898	45,6416	41,9231	38,8851	35,5632	33,4295	31,7946	30,4346	29,2463	28,1730	27,1789	26,2395	25,3365
27	55,4751	52,2152	49,6450	46,9628	43,1945	40,1133	36,7412	34,5736	32,9117	31,5284	30,3193	29,2266	28,2141	27,2569	26,3363
28	56,8918	53,5939	50,9936	48,2782	44,4608	41,3372	37,9159	35,7150	34,0266	32,6205	31,3909	30,2791	29,2486	28,2740	27,3362
29	58,3006	54,9662	52,3355	49,5878	45,7223	42,5569	39,0875	36,8538	35,1394	33,7109	32,4612	31,3308	30,2825	29,2908	28,3361

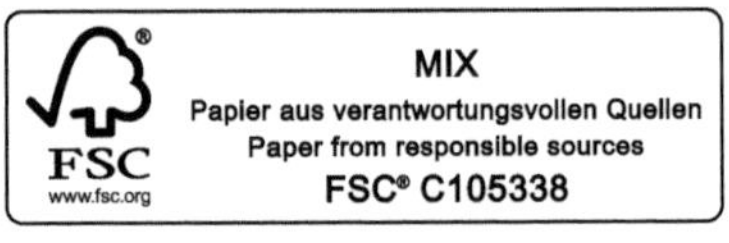

Printed by Books on Demand GmbH, Norderstedt / Germany